This book is a collective project drawing on the work of numerous individuals and organisations who have been campaigning to ensure that the National Health Service envisioned by Aneurin Bevan remains a reality. The contributors to this volume are:

Jacky Davis
Oliver Huitson
John Lister
Stewart Player
Allyson M. Pollock
David Price
Raymond Tallis
Charles West
David Wrigley

Keep Our NHS Public
London Health Emergency
NHS Consultants' Association
openDemocracy

For Aneurin Bevan and all those
who continue the fight for the NHS

NHS SOS

How the NHS Was Betrayed –

And How We Can Save It

Jacky Davis and Raymond Tallis, editors

ONEWORLD

A Oneworld Book

First published by Oneworld Publications 2013
Foreword copyright © 2013 Ken Loach
Introduction copyright © 2013 Raymond Tallis
'Breaking the Public Trust' copyright © 2013 John Lister
'Ready for Market' copyright © 2013 Stewart Player
'Parliamentary Bombshell' copyright © 2013 David Wrigley
'The Silence of the Lambs' copyright © 2013 Jacky Davis and David Wrigley
'The Failure of Politics' copyright © 2013 Charles West
'Hidden in Plain Sight' copyright © 2013 Oliver Huitson
'From Cradle to Grave' copyright © 2013 Allyson Pollock and David Price
'Stop Press: The Final Betrayal' copyright © 2013 David Wrigley and Jacky Davis
Afterword copyright © 2013 Jacky Davis and Raymond Tallis

ISBN: 978-1-78074-328-8
Ebook ISBN: 978-1-78074-329-5

Cover design by www.rooted-design.co.uk
Typeset by Tetragon, London
Printed and bound by CPI Group (UK) Ltd, Croydon, CR0 4YY

Oneworld Publications
10 Bloomsbury Street, London WC1B 3SR

Danger of abuse in the health service is not in the way that ordinary people use the service. Abuse is always at the point where private commercialism impinges on the service – where an attempt is made to marry the incompatible principles of private profit with public service.
The solution is to decrease the dependence on private enterprise.
A free health service is a triumphant example of the superiority of the principles of collective action and public initiative against the commercial principle of profit and greed.

Aneurin Bevan, *In Place of Fear*

The first guiding principle is this: maximise competition ... which is the primary objective.

Andrew Lansley

Contents

Foreword

Ken Loach

The reform of the National Health Service is, of course, to bring it back into the marketplace and degrade it back into making health care a commodity – so it's not reform at all.

If we don't understand that we've got to do everything, up to and including breaking the law, to defend the National Health Service, then we're finished.

First the words of a distinguished GP, then those of a former Liverpool dock worker. Across society, there is a realisation that the National Health Service is one of our greatest social achievements and that to keep it is an enormous political challenge.

This book is a weapon in that struggle. It shows how politicians of all parties, to a greater or lesser extent, have prepared the way for privatisation. It is a familiar pattern. The process in the health service began in the early 1980s, with the subcontracting of cleaning services. Why have we taken so long to respond? Are we so gullible that we believe politicians who say that the National Health Service is 'safe in their hands' when all the evidence is to the contrary?

In order to fight back, we need to understand the reasons for the attack on the NHS. This is an ideological issue. If it were simply a matter of finance, there are solutions to hand. There are billions of pounds in unpaid and uncollected taxes. Trillions, we are told, are kept off shore, beyond the reach of national governments. The wealth that is created by the work of ordinary people is siphoned off so that it cannot be used for the common good. If the political will to sustain a publicly funded health service existed, a way would be found.

It is a battle for ideas. To some, the drive for profit is a necessary discipline. Private business will see a need, provide the service in the most cost-effective way and make money in the process. Greed is good. When everyone pursues their own self-interest, so the theory goes, we all benefit.

Except that we don't. When the need can't yield a profit, the need goes unanswered. The health service and care services are full of examples of where people's requirements are not met. All who work there could fill many pages with stories. Further privatisation will widen the care gap and the so-called austerity programme diminishes every aspect of our life.

The resistance to this has been very weak. Those organisations that should be our first line of defence have let us down. The trades unions, crippled by Thatcher's government and abandoned by the Labour Party, have barely made an intervention. The Labour Party itself has followed the same path as its Tory predecessor in government. While trying to present a more humane face, it has continued the policies of privatisation and deregulation. When Labour adopted the slogan 'Labour

Means Business' it was not immediately apparent that it was meant literally.

This has left a political vacuum. Who puts forward the idea of working together for the common good? That we should be our brother's and sister's keeper? That we have the technology and the knowledge to provide a decent life for all but we are in the grip of an economic ideology that makes that impossible?

There is a fight-back taking place across Europe. Strikes and direct actions are seen in the countries hit hardest by mass unemployment and other consequences of economic failure. In Greece, France and Germany there are new political movements on the Left, putting forward alternatives. It has not happened yet in Britain. When people ask who they can vote for to defend the NHS, what do we tell them?

This book explains how current politicians have betrayed the principles of the NHS. In my view they are not worthy of our vote. If ever there was a time for there to be a broadly based movement, democratic and principled, which stood for the interests of the people against the demands of business and the politicians who speak for them, that moment is now.

List of Abbreviations and Acronyms

ACEVO	Association of Chief Executives of Voluntary Organisations
APMS	Alternative Provider Medical Services
ARM	Annual Representative Meeting
BMA	British Medical Association
BMJ	*British Medical Journal*
CQC	Care Quality Commission
CCG	Clinical Commissioning Group
CCP	Co-operation and Competition Panel
DoH	Department of Health
EGM	Extraordinary General Meeting
FESC	Framework for Procuring External Support for Commissioners
FT	Foundation Trust
GPC	General Practitioners Committee (of the BMA)
GPCos	GP Provider Companies
HMO	Health Maintenance Organisation
ICO	Integrated Care Organisation
IPA	Independent Practitioner Association
ISTC	Independent Sector Treatment Centre
KONP	Keep Our NHS Public
LHE	London Health Emergency

LIFT	Local Improvement Finance Trust
MCO	Managed Care Organisation
NAPC	National Association of Primary Care
NHSCB	NHS Commissioning Board
NLN	National Leadership Network
OFT	Office of Fair Trading
PCT	Primary Care Trust
PFI	Private Finance Initiative
PHO	Physician Hospital Organisation
PPG	Patient Participation Group
QIPP	Quality, Innovation, Productivity and Prevention
RGCP	Royal College of Psychiatrists
RCGP	Royal College of General Practitioners
RCM	Royal College of Midwives
RCN	Royal College of Nursing
RCP	Royal College of Physicians
RCOG	Royal College of Obstetricians and Gynaecologists
RCS	Royal College of Surgeons
SHA	Strategic Health Authority

Introduction

Raymond Tallis

The only thing necessary for the triumph of evil is that good men do nothing.

Edmund Burke

This book was conceived in desperate circumstances. In the summer of 2012 I attended the British Medical Association (BMA) Annual Representative Meeting (ARM) for the first time, in order to put forward a motion related to legislation of assisted dying. Three months earlier, Andrew Lansley's Health and Social Care Act had been passed in the House of Commons after a very protracted and bumpy ride (as Dr David Wrigley will describe). In the packed hall there was an attempt by one or two brave souls, including my co-editor, Dr Jacky Davis, to hold the BMA to account for its 'too little, too late' gestures towards opposing Lansley's bill. The debate was largely procedural, intended to make sure that no one was held responsible, and to deflect attention from the main issues. It was worse than uninspiring. Is this the best that the profession could do, I thought, when required to respond to the greatest threat to the health and well-being of the patients they are supposed to serve since the birth of the NHS?

On the second evening of the ARM, in deep despair, I decided to follow Jacky's advice to attend a fringe meeting at a pub near the conference centre. The contrast with the main event could not have been greater. There were about twenty people (half a dozen of them speakers) in a little back room, as opposed to the many hundreds in a beautifully appointed hall. The atmosphere was informal as opposed to the highly choreographed, closely scripted and minutely regulated show I had been sitting through earlier in the day. However, there was a more profound contrast. First, it was obvious that those who were present cared for the NHS and were enraged at what was going to happen to it. Second, the speeches, often given with the minimum of notes, were searching, well informed and impassioned. I had moved into another world, a world of which the medical profession was once a part.

The two hours I spent listening to the speakers was a crash course in what remained of principled medical politics. For the first time, I was able to see clearly how a toxic bill that few had foreseen and no one other than its proponents saw as desirable, even less necessary, had got on to the statute book. I felt that what I had learned in that small room should be more widely publicised. It seemed as if there were the makings of a book. I arranged for a few people to meet together for an early breakfast a couple of days later. And so began the process that led to *NHS SOS*.

This book is about the betrayal of the NHS – and of the people who depend on it for health and health care – by politicians, journalists, the unions and, perhaps most culpably, the leaders of the medical profession. Without the active collusion, passive acquiescence or incompetence of all of these players it would hardly have been possible for the Tories – who did not command a majority in Parliament – to have succeeded in getting Andrew Lansley's nightmare vision for the NHS enshrined in law. After all, prior to the 2010 election, the Tories had promised to defend the NHS not only from cuts to its budget but from the continuous redisorganisation that successive governments had inflicted on it over the preceding decades. This had been reaffirmed in the Coalition agreement: 'we will stop the top-down reorganisations of the NHS that have got in the way of patient care'.[1] Within a few months, the Coalition was boasting of the most radical shake-up of the service since 1948, the mother of all top-down reorganisations. This would be hugely destabilising and expensive,[2] at a time when, according to Sir David Nicholson, the NHS chief executive, the service would have to make £20 billion of efficiency savings in four years. Nor had any of the political parties given a hint in their manifestos that they would open up the NHS to wholesale privatisation. The impression from the Tory manifesto had been that the NHS would be financially protected – with increased spending year on year (a promise broken) – and otherwise left well alone. It was evident, however, that the plans had been in preparation a long time, though, as Nicholas Timmins has discovered, Lansley was banned from talking about them ahead of the election.[3]

Such blatant deception, such chutzpah, such contempt for the electorate, should have meant that the bill was doomed. While its passage to the statute book required (as Edmund Burke might have said) that good men should do nothing (or, with a few exceptions, very little), many other conditions were required, as described in the pages of this book. While each of these conditions was individually outrageous, the fact that they were able to come together to deliver the planned destruction of the NHS says something shocking – about the condition of the nation, the pervasiveness of corruption, the debased state of the national conversation about

matters of supreme importance, and the marginalisation of professionals who, when faced with the greatest threat for generations
to the institution and the values for which they claimed to stand,
in most cases preferred appeasement to confrontation, insisting
that the latter would be pointless.

While much of *NHS SOS* is about the failure of those who
should have sunk the bill – their failure to oppose it effectively, or
even with conviction – it is important not to forget that Andrew
Lansley's vision had its advocates. There have always been those
to whom the very idea of universal health care publicly funded,
publicly delivered and publicly accountable is repugnant, and would
remain so, even if it were shown that such services were the most
effective, cost-effective and popular mode of delivery. While attachment to the NHS has often been described as 'religious', hatred of
state-provided and state-funded services qualifies more fully for
the status of an article of passionate faith. The recent release of
the 1982 Cabinet papers shows how the 'mild-mannered, courte-
ous' Geoffrey Howe and his leader Margaret Thatcher dreamed
of 'dismantling the welfare state', accepting that this would be
'the end of the NHS'.[4] This caused a near riot in the Cabinet, not
because it was a wicked plan – which it was – but because it was
deemed 'politically toxic'. It took another thirty years of neoliberal
consensus thinking, as described by Stewart Player, for this to
become thinkable. As Ken Clarke said in 2008:

> Labour secretaries of state have got away with intro-
> ducing private sector providers into the NHS on a
> scale which would have led the Labour Party onto the
> streets in demonstration if a Conservative government
> had ever tried it. In the later 1980s I would have said

it is politically impossible to do what we are now doing.
I strongly approve.[5]

It was still unacceptable to the vast majority of those who provided and used public services. Moreover, in 2009 Andy Burnham,
Secretary of State for Health before the Coalition, made up for
some of the sins of his predecessors in the Labour administration
by making the NHS the service's 'preferred provider'. Consequently,
deceit was still necessary and, when the Lansley plan was eventually
brought into the open, it had to be spun. Doctors and patients were
to be reassured by politicians presenting the key aim of the bill as
putting the clinicians, notably GPs, in charge of health service budgets and what they were to be spent on, and, naturally, to 'increase
patient choice'. Just how far this is from the truth is set out in ter-
rifying detail in chapter 1 (Breaking the Public Trust) by John Lister,
and in chapter 7 (From Cradle to Grave) by Allyson M. Pollock and
David Price. That this spin was not adequately challenged, or even
critically examined, in the mass media is an outrage, as discussed by
Oliver Huitson in chapter 6 (Hidden in Plain Sight).

There were several potential sources of opposition to Lansley's
bill which, if fully mobilised, would have prevented its passage. These
were the medical profession, non-Tory politicians and the media.

The health care professions were best placed not only to understand
the true implications of Lansley's Health and Social Care Bill but
to influence public and parliamentary opinion against it. The Royal
College of Nursing made its hostility very clear but it was the doctors
whose views would carry most authority in the public mind. After all,
Lansley's assertion that his bill would put clinicians in the driving seat
would look rather strange if the majority of doctors said either that
they didn't believe him, or that they didn't want to be running NHS

budgets and were unqualified to commission services for populations. Unfortunately they, or at least their leaders, failed abjectly to oppose the bill effectively until it was too late, as Jacky Davis and David Wrigley reveal in chapter 4 (The Silence of the Lambs).

As Davis and Wrigley discuss, of the doctors who very much liked the idea of a service where they had control of the budget, some were motivated by altruism and others by self-interest. For some, to be blunt, the blatant systemic conflict of interest in providing services that they would themselves commission was embraced as an opportunity for personal enrichment. Greed was the spur. They were in a minority but they had disproportionate influence because they were pro-market and pro-GP commissioning and so had the government's ear. It would be interesting to know how much gold had been promised to stuff in the insatiable mouths of certain doctors. The rewards would come quickly. A survey in *Pulse* – the GPs' magazine – reported that by December 2012 over one-fifth of board members on clinical commissioning groups had financial interests in private health care providers; the BMJ put the number at more than one-third in March 2013.[6] Things are looking good for Dr Fat Cat.

Greed was not the main reason for the failure of many to question Lansley's bill before it was too late. After all, as I shall discuss, the most powerful, articulate and sustained opposition came from the Royal College of General Practitioners (RCGP), who looked at first as having the most to gain. No, there was a deeper malaise in the medical profession.

The political class has, over the last few decades, regarded doctors with increasingly open contempt. Instead of being respected as patients' advocates, and as having unique expertise in the best ways to care for patients and the best context in which that care might be delivered, they are portrayed as instinctively conservative, irrationally opposed to change, unable to see the need for it and obsessed by their own perceived self-interest. This has resulted in a progressive marginalisation of the role of doctors in the process of reshaping the services within which they work. Of course, each administration has found a sufficiency of useful idiots within the profession to act as cheerleaders for whatever idea crosses the mind of an ambitious Secretary of State. They are rewarded by flattery, first-class fares, gongs,[7] elevated office and financial opportunities. But the majority of doctors have gradually drifted to the margins of decision making, doing their best to work with whatever ill-thought-out ideas are foisted upon them by Whitehall.

I discussed the first twenty years of the marginalisation of the medical profession in *Hippocratic Oaths: Medicine and Its Discontents*, published just under a decade ago. Successive redisorganisations have further reduced the influence of the medical profession. In the late 1990s and early 2000s the opportunistic exploitation by politicians, most notably Alan Milburn, of medical scandals such as the problems with heart surgery in Bristol, the retention of organs at Alder Hey hospital and the mass murders by Harold Shipman, placed the profession on the back foot. Treating these episodes as symptomatic of a profession that was arrogant, dangerous and unaccountable was very damaging to its reputation.

Not everyone bought that image of the profession carefully fostered by politicians. As shown in poll after poll, doctors remain highly trusted – in contrast to politicians. Even so, the 'managerialism' in the NHS, which has progressed remorselessly since the first steps were taken in 1983 with the recommendations made by Roy Griffiths, has reduced many doctors to mere sessional functionaries. They are concerned to deliver on contracts narrowly defined, and less exercised by larger issues such as the context in which care is delivered and the health of the nation. Brian Jarman, in a recent article,[8] which should be required reading for anyone concerned about the health of the NHS, has examined the long-term effects of 'managerialism', most notably an imbalance of power between doctors and managers. Managers have considerable influence on the funding of hospital and other units, appointments to posts within hospitals and pay rises through the clinical excellence awards. They can refer doctors to the General Medical Council and there is no redress for groundless referral. Whistle-blowing doctors may be dismissed and, with their cards marked as troublemakers, they may find it difficult to obtain further employment in the NHS. (The Francis Report identified this as an important factor in the silence of doctors in the face of the wholesale abuse of patients in the Mid Staffordshire NHS Foundation Trust.) The Department of Health has spent very large sums of money on 'gagging agreements' for individuals dismissed from the service. A 'culture more of fear and of compliance, than of learning, innovation and enthusiastic participation in improvement' was identified in a report commissioned from Joint Commission International (an authoritative body on accrediting health care institutions).[9] Needless to say, this report was dismissed and deep-sixed by the Department of Health. David Nicholson regarded it as 'insignificant', which makes his very long tenure as CEO of the NHS easier to understand. It was exhumed only in response to a request under the Freedom of Information Act. Managers on the ground – many of whom are deeply committed to patient care – are themselves equally the victims of the 'top-down and bullying culture'.[10]

These trends have been exacerbated by the casualisation of the medical workforce and those pressures that Colin Leys identifies to make them become businessmen and -women, and which are described by Stewart Player in chapter 2 (Ready for Market).[11] 'Corporatising the NHS' requires instilling the corporate ethos into its workforce and replacing the fundamental idea (or at least ideal) of the professional as one who is bound by covenant to those he or she serves with versus a contract mediated through an ever-lengthening chain of intermediaries, each taking its cut. You are no longer the servant of the people who come to you for help or of the population from which they come, or answerable to the ideals of your profession. Your immediate loyalty is to a body whose primary oath is 'First Balance Your Books' or 'First Meet Your Targets' or 'First Satisfy Your Shareholders'. No wonder the Hippocratic Oath seems to have 'First Cover Your Ass' as the most important of its contemporary clauses. Troublemakers make trouble only for themselves. Gone is the consultant body that was the 'glue' that held hospitals together and defined their mission. And GPs who feel personal responsibility for the patients on his or her list are becoming less common. Stewart Player describes how the relationship between GPs and individual patients has been deliberately unpicked by health care policies over the last decade or more. Not everything is lost, however. Lord Owen is still correct when he asserts:

> The NHS is … a vocational service. It needs to retain within it a generosity of purpose, philosophical commitment and a one-to-one relationship with the individual patient.[12]

Nevertheless, the doctor as advocate for the vulnerable is in danger of becoming a thing of the past. This is excellent news for politicians for whom the professions, as an alternative source of authority, have always represented a threat[13] – second only to patients as a source of trouble. No wonder politicians like to spin advocacy for patients by the medical profession as self-interested. And, of course, there have been striking examples of such self-interest, most notably the BMA's opposition to the foundation of the NHS in 1948 and, more recently, the negotiation by its general practitioner body of a vastly enhanced salary, while handing over out-of-hours care to private providers.

Jacky Davis and David Wrigley's account (chapter 4) of the lamentable failure of the medical establishment to oppose Lansley's bill deals with the BMA's policy of 'critical engagement' with the Coalition – an overly generous description of what amounted to appeasement, which was maintained until it was far too late. The policy betrayed either a fatal political naivety or a cynical decision to back the bill while pretending otherwise. While this was pathetic, it was less shocking than the way in which the BMA acted with little regard to the views of its members. What is more, it failed to work together with other professional bodies such as the medical royal colleges to put up a united front. It seems unlikely that the bill would have survived the opposition of a united profession.

The royal colleges' performance individually and collectively (in the feeble body the Academy of Medical Royal Colleges) was also dismal. Indeed, the Royal College of Physicians (RCP) was stung into action only by the determined efforts of a few activists who called for an Extraordinary General Meeting (EGM) at which the bill was rejected. The leaders of the RCP found this so traumatic that one of their first subsequent actions was to propose an increase in the number of fellows necessary to call an EGM in future![14] In the light of Davis and Wrigley's account of the muted response of the Academy of Medical Royal Colleges in early 2012, it was exasperating to be told of the Academy's concerns about the implications of the Health and Social Care Act a year after it had been passed, as if they had suddenly discovered the plans for mass privatisation of the NHS.[15]

The impotence of the profession, or its representative bodies, and the feebleness of its leadership (with one or two extraordinary exceptions) should not occasion surprise. The medical establishment had scarcely noticed – or if they had, done nothing to oppose – the trends over the previous decades that I have just described, which were making it easier for politicians to ignore them. The failure to see that Lansley's bill was a threat to their fundamental purpose was myopia as usual. They seem not to have grasped that their mission to improve the quality of doctoring and maintain the highest standards of patient care is not deliverable within a political framework that undermines it. It is unlikely that the royal colleges' well-meaning reports would attract much attention from the senior executives of UnitedHealthcare, Serco or Virgin Care.[16] The image that comes to mind is of a series of ridge tents pitched on an avalanche.

The inspiring exception to the mild-mannered protests of the royal colleges (concerned not to upset anyone or threaten their charitable status by being accused of being 'political') and the BMA's advocacy of 'critical engagement' (not exactly an adequate response to threatened destruction of everything you are supposed to stand for) was the Royal College of General Practitioners. Their courageous leader Dr Clare Gerada maintained to the very end that the bill would 'cause irreparable damage to patient care and jeopardise the NHS'.[17] The story of Gerada's lonely opposition should shame those who kept mum, whatever their reason. Had she been supported by the other powerful medical bodies in her call for the bill to be dropped, then 'Dr Lansley's Monster' (as the *British Medical Journal* called it[18]) might well have assumed its rightful place in the dustbin of history.

I have focused on the betrayal by the medical profession but there were other parties who failed to mount an effective opposition to Lansley's bill. The other health care unions – which would be an interesting study in themselves – while they were clearly opposed to the bill, did not manage to make themselves heard. They were, of course, in a weaker position than the royal colleges because their clearly expressed views could more easily be dismissed as self-interested. But there were two other players: the media and the politicians. I want to say something briefly about each.

First, the media. As Oliver Huitson demonstrates, with a few honourable exceptions (most notably Polly Toynbee and her colleagues at the *Guardian*, the online openDemocracy and, from time to time, the *Mail* group of newspapers), there was a failure in many print and broadcast media to grasp and communicate the implications of Lansley's proposed changes. The mantras of 'putting the patient at the heart of the NHS' and placing most of the NHS budget (variously quantified as £60 billion and £80 billion annual expenditure) in the hands of GPs was reported and repeated endlessly. In fact, as Pollock and Price make clear in chapter 7, the most important budgetary consequence of the bill would be to place both commissioning and provision of services in the hands of private providers, concealing from public scrutiny the way the health care budget was being spent and, of course, distancing the Secretary of State from responsibility for an increasingly privatised service. Just how little awareness there was of the serious implications of Lansley's bill is reflected in the findings of an Ipsos MORI poll conducted in February 2012, just as the battles in the House of Lords were reaching their climax, in that only 22 per cent of those surveyed regarded the NHS as the most important issue facing Britain – a long way behind immigration.[19]

Second, the politicians. The Tories in opposition deceived the public about their plans for the NHS but at least their aims were in accordance with their ideological preference for private over public provision or, failing that, marketised public services. They were being true to their unprincipled principles. As Stewart Player shows in chapter 2, Labour were most culpable; in particular Alan Milburn, whose ultimate ambition – not made clear to those who had elected him – was to make the NHS 'a kitemark attached to the institutions and activities of purely private providers'.[20] The Tories were entirely justified in claiming (when they were not describing the bill as 'revolutionary') that their proposals were a realisation of a plan dreamed up by the neoliberal wing of the Labour Party; that they were finishing Labour's dirty work for it. Lansley's destruction of the NHS has been a long time in the making.

This left the Lib Dems, who are the focus of Charles West's insider account in chapter 5 (A Failure of Politics). Without their support it is inconceivable that a minority Conservative government could have got the bill through. What is more, that support was in the face of opposition from their own grassroots membership, who, as West makes clear, were deceived and outmanoeuvred by their leaders. Nick Clegg's wavering and confusion – due in part to his initial careless inattention to the bill and its implications – is shocking. It was probably not a symptom of the corruption that comes from power – it was too quick for that – but perhaps the equally dangerous corrupting effect of impotence, not too different from that which had been seen in the Labour Party's reinvention of itself, and betrayal of its principles, in the years out of office.

One of the great mysteries that West tries to make sense of is Shirley Williams's defence of the bill at a crucial moment, having earlier made plain her opposition to its core features. It is tragic that Williams's capitulation, which would have such malign consequences, might be the most important decision in her distinguished career of public service.

Let me end this overture by addressing several questions that may be crossing the reader's mind.

First, *is the bill really as destructive as some have painted it?* Does it matter who provides health care, so long as it is of a high standard and is free at the point of need? The answers to these questions are to be found in chapter 7 in particular, where Allyson M. Pollock and David Price spell out the consequences of an unravelling NHS. It will take some time for these consequences to unfold but once they have done so, and it is realised that something catastrophic has happened, it will be more difficult to reverse the changes. No administration will be able to buy out the private sector and return the NHS to public ownership or recreate a coherent service from the fragments in the hands of dozens of private providers. Think how, after many years of chaos, renationalising the railways was a financial impossibility. We must act urgently.

Second, *is the NHS worth saving?* On the most disinterested assessments, the NHS is both efficient and effective and is currently enjoying a very high level of approval ratings – over 90 per cent – by those who use it. A report by The Commonwealth Fund assessing quality, efficiency, access to care, equity and healthy lives in different health systems in seven industrialised countries, was published in June 2010, just before Lansley's plans were sprung on the nation. It rated the NHS very highly on quality of, and access to, care; it was top (above, for example, Australia and the Netherlands) on efficiency.[21] By contrast the US – the inspiration for much of Lansley's thinking – was a dismal last in all measures. Even more tellingly, a report published in January 2013 found that the US, which devotes a staggering 18 per cent of its economy to health spending (double the percentage of the UK), is at or near the bottom in measures of health and life expectancy in sixteen economically wealthy countries.[22]

The NHS, however, does have its problems. The shocking findings of the Francis Inquiry into the neglect of patients at the Mid Staffordshire NHS Foundation Trust indicate the scale of such problems in some places.[23] But the Health and Social Care Act 2012 will not solve them; rather it will make them worse. We may anticipate resources siphoned off into the pockets of private providers, and the atomisation of services. This will be associated with the fragmentation of health care into discrete functions provided by individuals whose primary loyalty must be to the company. Those who blow the whistle on bad, negligent, dangerous and unethical practice in a privatised NHS will face even greater risks to their personal prospects. Indeed, it is the quasi-marketisation of the NHS, with desperately competitive management and 'de-professionalised' professionals, and the introduction of much-lauded 'private sector disciplines' and 'private sector values' that lay behind much of the awfulness of what went on in the Mid Staffordshire Trust. And the events at Winterbourne (hidden from) View, where patients were abused at the per capita cost to the taxpayer of £150,000 a year, hardly demonstrate the humanising influence of the market in health care.

Third, *why rake over the past?* The answer is straightforward. If we do not examine and come to understand the context that led to Lansley's act, we shall not be able to reverse the most toxic parts of it. Most of this book focuses on that context: deceitful politicians with their weasel words; a demoralised, supine or 'de-professionalised' profession; and failings of the media in their duty to inform. It is not enough to be tough on Lansley: we need to be tough on the causes of Lansley so that what happened in 2012, for which the way was prepared in the preceding decades, can never be repeated. *NHS SOS* has been written in the belief that effective opposition requires clear diagnosis of the pathological background and aetiology of the Health and Social Care Act 2012, in particular the corruption of the political process that permitted a drive towards universal privatisation without a political mandate.

Fourth, *can there be effective opposition?* Isn't it all too late? We believe that there is room for hope. The most pernicious parts of Lansley's act can be removed without yet a further reorganisation. Reinstatement of the duties of the Secretary of State for Health and of the NHS as the preferred provider for services would limit many of the damaging effects of Lansley's dream. It is heartening, and reassuring, that this view is shared with as astute and experienced a politician as Lord Owen, who has tabled a bill to this effect.[24]

Fifth and finally, *what can we do to create effective opposition?* This is the theme of the Afterword by Jacky Davis and myself. It is based on the collective wisdom of many of our contributors and we hope it will motivate readers to act.

So, the battle is engaged. It is of supreme importance. The NHS was created at a time of great austerity (much more severe than that which the bankers and their neoliberal friends have inflicted on the people of this country) and belongs to an era in which each of us recognises that we share the vulnerability of all. We must not allow this jewel in the crown of the welfare state to be destroyed by those whose rapacious self-interest has rendered them unable to comprehend any notion of the public good or public service. If the corporate raiders succeed, some of us will die from lack of care, many more will undergo unnecessary suffering due to ill health,[25] and more still will experience financial ruin. This seems a high price to pay for making the world pleasing to hedge fund managers and multinational companies, whose interests are increasingly dominant in the corrupted parliamentary processes shaping every aspect of our lives.

If Percy Shelley were alive today, he would have to admit that it is not the poets but the Fortune 500 who are the 'unacknowledged legislators of the world'. It is perhaps more than a little ambitious to hope that we might be able to change this. However, foiling politicians' plans to turn the NHS into a lucrative industry – something for which there is no political mandate – that will provide fewer and worse services at greater cost is something that lies within our powers.[26]

1

BREAKING THE PUBLIC TRUST

John Lister

All politicians lie, just like the rest of us, only more so.

Polly Toynbee

It could be said that the National Health Service as we know it was abolished in April 2013, just three months short of its sixty-fifth birthday. This was not a peaceful process. There is no consensus behind the highly contentious Health and Social Care Act 2012, which after a belated, lengthy tussle through Parliament eventually passed to set the new framework.

The old NHS is being painfully put down, rather than pensioned off – but there is some hope for reviving it, if the public comes together to fight for it. It is consistently high in the public's affections. When David Cameron's Coalition Government took office it had received a decade of record investment, allowing it to meet ambitious targets to cut waiting times and improve care, and was achieving record levels of public satisfaction. It was not broken, and did not need fixing.

Indeed, far from fixing or improving the NHS, the massive unwanted Tory 'reforms' have a very different purpose, enabling profit-seeking private companies and non-profit social enterprises to emerge and challenge for a growing share of health budgets, win contracts – and find inclusion on a new, lightly regulated register of so-called 'Qualified Providers'. Meanwhile, public sector (NHS) providers are being continuously cut and squeezed into downsizing, mergers, centralisation and closures. Cynical 'reconfiguration' plans being driven through across England mean only a reduced number of short-staffed, demoralised, overloaded 'centralised' units will remain, covering only those services that the private sector does not wish to provide.

The eclipse of the public sector delivery of health care is no accident. In place of what was for many years a unified system, one that publicly provided a comprehensive range of services to the whole population on the basis of clinical need rather than ability to pay,[1] the NHS has been quite deliberately reduced by the Health and Social Care Act 2012 to little more than a fund of taxpayers' money through which services are purchased from a variety of providers. This continued role for public funding has – for the time being at least – allowed health ministers to insist that the proposals are 'not privatisation', since treatment will still be free at point of use, despite the fact that the provider of elective and community services is increasingly likely to be a private company or social enterprise.[2]

Previous Conservative governments have not scrupled to reorganise health services that once were free at point of use, so that very large numbers of patients are now subject to charges for their care. The most obvious examples have been the disappearance of NHS dentistry for many, and soaring charges even for those who can still access NHS dental services; the removal of free eye tests and almost all free provision of NHS spectacles;

and, of course, the biggest privatisation of them all so far: the effective privatisation of social care.

Under Margaret Thatcher's so-called 'community care' reforms (following the 1988 Griffiths Report), long-term care of the elderly, which had previously been financed through the NHS and through social security entitlements, was in 1993 removed from the brief of the NHS and handed over to local council social service departments, where it has remained subject to means-tested charges. As a result, each year thousands of people have to sell their houses to pay for care that once was free. A majority of older people in care homes now pay most of the costs of their own care, while almost all home help and domiciliary services for the frail elderly have been privatised. Councils levy charges based on a person's income and assets: the charges are being constantly driven upwards by central government funding cuts, even as eligibility for support has been reduced to those with the most extreme needs, leaving others to fend for themselves.[3]

FLASHBACK

The 2010 White Paper by then Health Secretary Andrew Lansley, cynically entitled 'Equity and excellence: Liberating the NHS', began with an explicit commitment to enforce the target of £20 billion in cost savings to be achieved by the NHS by 2014.

The subsequent Health and Social Care Act 2012 is a major turning point. When the NHS was founded in 1948 it represented a historic, qualitative leap forward over any previous system, superseding the crisis-ridden 'mixed economy' of health care that had preceded the war and which quickly proved unable to meet demand. Today, it is being replaced by a new 'mixed economy' of health care, a change that the public has never called for or supported, and a system that will cost more but be less efficient and deliver less care. Driven not by evidence but by ideology, the Tories have reinvented the flat tyre.

More or less the only people celebrating the passing of Andrew Lansley's controversial bill in March 2012 were in the private sector, itching to get their hands on a larger slice of the £100 billion health budget in England that now is still largely spent with public sector services.[4] The Health and Social Care Act opened the way for that to change.

To make room for a private health sector that has lamentably failed to develop any viable market for its own expansion, it has been necessary to cut the public sector provision, and to create a new competitive health care market in those services that the private companies see as profitable – provided they are backed by government funding.

To do this, the existing structures of the NHS had to be extensively reorganised. Within months of taking office Lansley, as the Coalition's first Health Secretary, jettisoned his own party's previous public pledges of 'no more top-down reorganisation', and drew up a 354-page bill that was substantially larger than Nye Bevan's 1946 act which set up the NHS. While Lansley repeatedly insisted that his enormous and complex bill proposed a plan for evolution rather than revolution, the NHS chief executive Sir David Nicholson was marginally more honest when he admitted that the change was so big it was 'visible from space'.[5]

CUTBACK

This wholesale reorganisation of the NHS required other abrupt policy reversals by Lansley and by Cameron. From 2006 onwards they (with other Tory MPs) had posed as allies, even champions, of several local campaigns against hospital cuts and closures. Then, in the run-up to the 2010 general election they promised to impose a 'moratorium' on further closures of A&E and maternity services and to increase NHS spending in real terms year by year.[6] They even made special commitments to safeguard a few hospitals close to Tory Party electoral interests, such as Chase Farm Hospital in Enfield and Queen Mary's in Sidcup. However, after the election such pledges and the brief moratorium were swiftly dropped. Within months the changes were felt at Queen Mary's, with the process of rundown accelerated and its A&E closed. The drive to axe Chase Farm was also renewed. These and similar cuts were part of the wave of cutbacks that have been unleashed since Lansley's 2010 White Paper launched an unprecedented and sustained cash squeeze on the NHS. Hospitals and other health trusts were required to generate cost savings of more than 4 per cent per year, year after year, a cumulative target of £20 billion – with actual cuts dressed up as 'efficiency savings'.

Cuts, closures and rationing of public sector services run hand in glove with privatisation and the creation of a new market for health care. The aim is to scale down public providers, downgrade and discredit public services, and strengthen the position of private companies such as Serco and Virgin who have their eyes on winning contracts to deliver services, especially in primary care and community health.

It's no accident therefore that prominent among the cuts have been moves by growing numbers of local commissioners to exclude more and more elective treatments and operations from the list of services available on the NHS.[7] Where the NHS will no longer fund a treatment, such as a hip or knee replacement, or hernia and varicose vein operations, the patient has an invidious choice: go private – and pay up for treatment that once was available to all who needed it free of charge – or go without.

This rationing of health care (which has the effect of restrict-ing access to services sweepingly dismissed as of 'limited clinical benefit' to only those who can pay) was one of the extensive series of proposals for cost-cutting outlined in a report written by the giant multinational consultancy McKinsey and Company and commissioned by the Labour Government in 2009.[8] In public ministers always denied that rationing was under discussion, even after Essex became the first of many authorities to explore the possibilities of using rationing and exclusions to save money in the dying days of the Labour Government. More recently, Coalition ministers have been the ones claiming innocence – even as they tighten the financial screw on local commissioners.

To drive through cutbacks and unpopular policies on the scale put forward by the Health and Social Care Act 2012 requires dilut-ing of the already limited accountability of local NHS bodies and service providers. Starting in April 2013, primary care trusts (PCTs) and strategic health authorities (SHAs), which once commissioned and planned health care on behalf of local and regional populations in England, were replaced by 'local' bodies that are anything but public – over two hundred clinical commissioning groups (CCGs).

In theory the CCGs are controlled by local GPs, and this has been the main argument used by ministers to defend them. But from the outset it was clear that this was unlikely to happen in any meaningful way. Most GPs remained resolutely opposed to the Health and Social Care Act, and would not step forward for a role invented to support it. For the most part they recognised that if they were forced into the role of commissioners, they would have to take the blame for imposing cutbacks and the rationing of care to their own patients, which were integral elements of the reform package. Some also recognised that GPs would have little day-to-day control over running their local CCG. As clinicians with a caseload of patients, most GPs lack the time, energy and inclination to take on a major strategic management job involving a nine-figure budget, or for planning services in much wider areas than their own practice.

A handful of well-meaning but misguided idealists have hung in and engaged with the development of the new CCGs,[9] but the involvement of doctors has been mostly limited to a group of willing 'reformers', many with an eye to potential personal gain and increased local influence available under the new scheme.

In practice local CCGs will function almost entirely through their small, largely self-selected executive boards, many of which barely trouble to consult the wider community of GPs in their area before taking far-reaching decisions about the provision of health care. For instance, in north-west London, the primary care trusts (acting together as 'NHS NW London') hatched a plan in 2012 to close four A&E units and wider plans involving the closure of more than one-quarter of the acute beds, with the loss of over five thousand jobs, many of them clinical staff. This was an astonishing change in health care services for the community, but the PCT announced a public consultation on the A&E closures one day, and almost the next claimed that the plans were supported by all of the north-west London shadow CCGs. Few GPs outside the magic circle of board members were fully aware of the proposals, and none of those who were aware of them had been asked to register their views.[10]

THE OPPOSITE OF DEVOLUTION

The CCGs report to a newly created, national body that is neither public nor locally based – the NHS Commissioning Board now known as 'NHS England' – and its twenty-seven secretive subdivisions, called local area teams.[11] The NHS England Board gets to vet the constitution of every CCG, retaining the right to intervene in a CCG's activities, including the ability to force a merger with another CCG or force a change of the CCG's chief executive if the CCG does not fall in line. NHS England will impose tight cash limits on the CCGs. It will set detailed guidelines on how CCGs must work, defining the limited scope they have to decide basic things such as who should provide local services. The goal, it seems, from reading the legislation, is to have decisions that were once in the hands of the doctors, and then in the hands of PCTs, framed and controlled from above.

Given the pressures on GPs, implementing the reforms was always going to be delegated to a management team. For the past couple of years, a number of PCTs had begun to establish 'referral management centres', which were intended to help cut health care costs by reducing referrals to hospital. GP referral letters increasingly went not to the chosen hospital but to a referral management centre, some of which were run for profit by private companies. The centres would second-guess the decision of the GP and patient, without knowing anything about them, suggesting that a cheaper alternative treatment was more appropriate. The referral would be sent back to the GP – making a complete travesty of 'patient choice'. *Pulse* magazine, whose readers are mainly GPs, found that around one in eight referrals were being 'bounced back' in this way, even before the latest financial squeeze.[12] This centralised model is likely to be extended further by NHS England, looking over the decisions of CCGs with an eye to cost containment and efficiency.

There is also the fear that in more and more cases CCGs' own management teams will be steered by private sector management consultants. In the first instance the CCG commissioning support services (many of them former primary care trust and strategic health authority staff) have been organised by NHS England. But by

2016 'commissioning support services' must be 'externalised', that is, put out to tender,[13] offering rich pickings for the management consultants – McKinsey, Ernst & Young, PricewaterhouseCoopers and Capita, to name a few of the usual suspects. The handful of GPs who have taken a spot on CCG boards are trapped by cash limits, decisions imposed by the outgoing PCTs, and by the outside forces of referral management centres and commissioning support services; they are bullied by NHS England and unlikely to be able to 'reform from within'. A CCG cannot even claim to have any popular mandate or support, since CCGs were set up without any public consultation or involvement. The process makes a transparent nonsense of Andrew Lansley's assurance of 'no decision to be taken about me, without me'.

In fact, coupled with the budget squeeze, the Health and Social Care Act guarantees that almost every decision on the development and configuration of services is now being taken without any regard to the views of local people, or even in the teeth of popular opposition. Consultation exercises about the future of the NHS and local commissioning have been a farce, and any strong expression of public outrage at the changes has been brushed aside, with only sketchy, tokenistic attempts to address local concerns over the closure of hospitals and A&Es.

The most outrageous example of this, of course, has been the use of the draconian powers of the 'unsustainable provider regime' in the case of South London Healthcare Trust, which was facing massive financial problems. A special administrator was named, but, finding it impossible to lay their hands on sufficient cash savings within the trust, the administrator opted to spread the pain and axe a successful and popular neighbouring hospital in Lewisham. This was despite huge local protests and opposition from the local council, community organisations, over ninety hospital consultants who signed detailed critiques of the administrator's proposals and the Lewisham CCG itself.[14]

END OF TRUST

The PCTs are not the only part of the NHS as we know it that are being abolished by the Health and Social Care Act. NHS trusts are to be abolished too. Until now, NHS trusts – whether they are providers of hospital services, mental health, community or ambulance services – have held their board meetings in public, published board papers and had an obligation to consult on major changes. But under the act, any NHS trusts that have not yet gained foundation trust status are required to take steps to do so by 2014. Foundation trusts are run as not-for-profit businesses ('independent Public Benefit Corporations').[15] Their boards are 'free' to meet in secret, can choose not to publish their board papers and can take far-reaching decisions with reference only to the national regulator. Most foundation trusts have taken full advantage of this freedom to be more secretive and withhold information that has previously been in the public domain.[16] Lansley's plan is to go much further and remove the foundation trusts from the NHS balance sheet altogether, effectively completing the process of privatisation.[17]

The establishment of foundation trusts in 2004 had signalled a substantial break in the accountability of NHS hospital managers. Previously, managers had reported to the Secretary of State, who reported on to Parliament, allowing MPs to raise questions of concern relating to their local hospitals. But as soon as the first hospitals were converted into foundation trusts, they were no longer accountable either to NHS management structures or directly to government.[18] Only the regulator, Monitor, itself a body dominated from the outset by management consultants, many of them former employees of McKinsey (or contractors still employed by McKinsey), had powers to intervene.[19]

We now know that those powers to intervene were very limited, and the level of regulation was grossly inadequate. A hard-hitting report, issued early in 2013 by the Commons Public Accounts Committee, exposed the impotence of Monitor's attempts to intervene to dissuade the board of Peterborough and Stamford Hospitals Foundation Trust from proceeding with what has emerged as a disastrously expensive £310 million contract for a privately funded hospital in Peterborough.[20] Two letters from Monitor to the board warning against the expense of the project were ignored, not only by the board but also by the strategic health authority, the Department of Health, the Treasury, and Health Minister Andy Burnham. All of these parties signed off on what has become a £2 billion, 612-bed hospital project that has plunged the foundation trust into a massive, unpayable deficit, equivalent to one-quarter of its annual turnover.[21] Further, the calamitous failure of Mid Staffordshire NHS Foundation Trust to deliver adequate standards of health care has been well documented by the two Francis Reports, underlining the feeble efforts of the Health Care Commission, the forerunner to today's Care Quality Commission (CQC) to check on the quality of care in the area. Monitor also rubber-stamped Mid Staffordshire's application for foundation trust status after minimal scrutiny, overlooking the desperate cuts in staffing that were necessary in order to wipe out the £10 million deficit and achieve a balanced budget – usually with 'surpluses' built in to pay for the development of their services – as required for foundation status.[22]

While these failures of scrutiny and regulation remain unresolved, showing the weaknesses of the current system of regulation of foundation trusts, the Health and Social Care Act 2012 establishes an even more fundamental accountability gap: the provision that ends the direct duty of the Secretary of State to provide health services to England's communities and passing this responsibility to the new NHS Commissioning Board, accountable to no one in government.[23]

HOSPITALS TREATED AS BUSINESSES

Already the early symptoms of a commercial market are emerging. NHS foundation trusts and hospital trusts are no longer regarded under the law as public services, but as profit-seeking businesses, along the lines of a Tesco, United Biscuits or Barclays. When NHS trusts and foundations generate modest 'surpluses' – as required in order to meet government targets – these are viewed almost as though they were profits, even though, unlike profits, NHS surpluses cannot be pocketed by shareholders.[24, 25]

Indeed, mergers between foundation and hospital trusts are now investigated as *commercial* transactions by the Office of Fair Trading (OFT). Even cash-saving reconfigurations of services are probed for their impact on competition and local health markets by the so-called Co-operation and Competition Panel (CCP), which was set up by Labour in 2009 and has been utilised eagerly by the Coalition as part of the quiet efforts to transform the NHS into a commercial market for health care.[26] From the beginning, the core assumption among CCP (and OFT) staff has been that competition and choice of providers is *always* better for patients and that it is a means for securing better 'health care' value for money. However, there is a marked lack of evidence to support this pro-market view.

In early 2013 the Coalition moved to lay far-reaching additional regulations before Parliament, setting out how the Health and Social Care Act should be implemented, which threatens to further tighten the screws. The parliamentary procedure used rarely results in any explicit discussion, debate or vote, and ministers expected that, with little challenge made to them, they would become law at the end of March. However, the resistance and public awareness have been far greater than expected, and as this book goes to press the final outcome of the now revised regulations is not yet certain.

The new regulations, under Section 75 of the act, flew in the face of Lansley's repeated assurances that GPs, through their role in the CCGs, would not be required to open up local services to competition. Instead, they would compel CCGs to either put health services out to tender or open them up to 'Any Qualified Provider'.[27] In addition Monitor was to be given greater powers to step in where it deems the new rules have been broken. The regulations also set out to prevent any attempt to treat existing NHS organisations as 'preferred providers'. Instead they sought to put in place a 'right to establish and provide services' by any party – a right that exists in the EU, that has resulted in rich opportunities for private health providers to take on the least complex and most profitable patient services. CCGs that opt to use the 'Any Qualified Provider' provision of Section 75 must accept any provider that has been approved by the Care Quality Commission (CQC) and Monitor, and include them on the list of providers offered to local patients. But no explicit guidelines exist on the qualifications required for a provider to satisfy the so far 'light touch' regulation of the CQC and Monitor. It appears that the only qualification necessary is financial solvency.

As this demonstrates, from day one of their full operation, the entirety of the legal and government pressure on CCGs is directed to ensure that they open up as many services as possible for private providers. The marginally less damaging system of competitive tendering – in which the CCGs at least get to exercise some control, in vetting bids and choosing which providers should be trusted to care for local patients – is far more time consuming for many of the resource-strapped doctors on CCGs. In this way the Section 75 regulations nudge CCGs towards the worse option: the chaotic marketplace of 'Any Qualified Provider'.

Behind these increasingly overt uses of home-grown competition law stands the tacit, looming threat of the EU. The EU's competition laws are designed to help ensure that once any service is privatised, there is no way for the state to take it back into public ownership. This would stand in the way of the 'sacred right' of the private sector to compete to deliver services that entrepreneurs consider to be profitable. Better yet, the private sector can cash in on public funding during the transition, without sharing any of the financial risks inflicted on the public sector providers.

MAKING A PROFIT

Whether the senior managers of public sector hospitals like it or not, these new laws and regulations mean that they are being forced to act more and more on the logic of private hospitals and commercial businesses. The first line of attack in this crusade has been to look for ways to duck out of providing services – such as A&E – which do not offer guaranteed returns. Seeking to pass muster and qualify for foundation status, as required by the Health and Social Care Act 2012, NHS trusts including London's Whittington Hospital Trust are heeding the advice of Monitor to find savings by cutting back or closing down those services that do not contribute positively to the financial balance sheet.[28] Cutting back on A&E is a way to drive wider cuts in other services.

Another twist has been added by Section 165 of the Health and Social Care Act, which specifically removed the previous 'cap' on the amount of private medical treatment that could be undertaken by foundation trusts. Previously, they had been limited to private income no greater (as a proportion of turnover) than their income when they shifted from hospital status to foundation status. The concession had been reluctantly incorporated into the legislation that established foundation trusts in 2003 by Labour Health Secretary Alan Milburn, in an effort to placate the concerns among several backbench Labour MPs that the changes to the NHS were a back-door move to privatisation. The financial caps, if not the concerns, have now been swept away. The new formula allows foundation trusts to make up to half of their annual total revenue from private medicine.[29]

As a result, some foundations, especially the wealthier and more prestigious specialist and teaching hospitals based in London, are beginning to boost their income from private treatment – it's the only way possible in the squeezed and frozen NHS. With commissioners seeking to meet their financial targets by reducing hospital referrals year by year, new providers trying to slice off an ever larger share of the budgets for elective treatment, and the standard tariff of payments for each item of treatment set to fall each year for the next several years (yielding less income for the same work), there is no escape from decline – for as long as trusts depend exclusively on public sector funding. The Health and Social Care Act formula opens just one possible route to raise additional revenue – and that is through private medicine. As a result, NHS patients in these hospitals are inevitably transformed into less desirable, second-class customers as compared with the lure of lucrative cash payments from wealthy patients from home or abroad.

PURE FINANCIAL INCOMPETENCE

However much trusts and foundations are compelled to act like businesses, many of them are saddled with the enormous costs of a policy that could only have been imposed on the public sector. The culprit is the Private Finance Initiative, or PFI.

As a tactic, PFI was developed in the 1980s and 1990s, gaining steam under Prime Minister John Major, as a means to finance big infrastructure projects in Britain. Hospitals were among the most profitable targets of the scheme. Rather than having the government build and maintain these structures, a for-profit outfit would get a contract to do so, then lease the new buildings to the NHS trust, together with a contract for support services, for a period of twenty-five to thirty years.

Initially, politicians claimed that making use of private capital would somehow be cheaper than using Treasury funding, or government borrowing. This was quickly discredited. But for politicians, the appeal was not just in these phantom cost savings; they were lured by the prospect of securing new buildings in their constituencies more quickly and apparently off the books of public borrowing. For those who were willing to ignore the downsides, it was a win-win.

It was even claimed that the private sector would enter into some form of 'partnership' with the NHS, although as a partnership PFI has been compared to a deal in which two men own a cow: one mucks it out, feeds and milks it, and the other sells the milk ... and pockets the cash. Any self-respecting private business would have laughed these 'business cases' out of court and rejected the notion outright.[30]

The Tories tried but never managed to persuade major investors to sign up for any of their proposed PFI-funded hospital projects. The fear at the time was that individual NHS trusts might go broke and be unable to pay off the amount owing. That issue was resolved with the arrival of New Labour. After Tony Blair took office, the 'New Labour' Government passed legislation exempting the private sector from this risk, thereby guaranteeing a long-term, stable profit stream coveted by corporate accountants. The floodgates were opened. In the deluge that followed over one hundred NHS PFI schemes were signed off.

Most of the NHS PFI schemes are now operational, with projects valued at £11 billion. The contracts stipulate that payments on the leases are index-linked, rising a minimum of 2.5 per cent each year. With most leases running for thirty years or more, the Treasury estimates that they will cost £65 billion – and potentially much more, if inflation continues above target.[31]

These steadily rising bills have to be paid by trusts facing a continual decline in income, as referrals are squeezed down and tariffs are reduced. Another problem is that many PFI hospitals tried to hold down costs by reducing the numbers of beds they provided – with the first wave of PFI hospitals cutting bed numbers by one-quarter or more, which means they lack the capacity to deal with peaks in demand. The buildings are inflexible, unaffordable and, in many cases, despite the glossy façades, uncomfortable and poorly designed for staff to work in and for patients.

Five years after the meltdown in the banking sector triggered a massive financial crisis and brought a halt to the expansion and improvement of public services, the taxpayer still owns some of the banks that were most active in exploiting the profits from PFI. Yet these same banks are still milking hefty payments from troubled NHS trusts. In addition, according to a European Services Strategy Unit report, as many as seventy PFI contracts are now owned by companies based off shore, also meaning that they pay no tax to HM Revenue and Customs.[32]

As the financial straitjacket has been tightened, PFI has been at the centre of the financial problems of a growing number of trusts. In February 2012 seven NHS trusts in England, including the one in Peterborough, were granted access to a new £1.5 billion bailout fund set up by Andrew Lansley – a move designed to leave the main structure of PFI intact. To qualify for the money, the trusts had to jump through hoops and show that they had plans for cuts and efficiency savings.

The pattern remains clear: NHS services and non-PFI hospitals will be cut, cut and cut again to ensure that the flow of cash and profits to PFI consortia and their shareholders remains protected. In south-east London the first PFI-damaged hospital trust has been declared insolvent and has been carved up by a special administrator, along with the closure of most services at neighbouring Lewisham – all with minimal public consultation or right of appeal. Money is no object: £200 million of debts have been written off, and PFI payments subsidised, in a plan that will cost a staggering £700 million or more, and undermine services across south-east London.[33]

But the first PFI trust to suffer this indignity might well have been Peterborough and Stamford Hospitals NHS Foundation Trust, which has repeatedly hit national headlines as its massive and costly PFI scheme lurched predictably out of control. Other trusts with major PFI-fuelled deficits are also being scrutinised, including Mid Yorkshire Hospitals, University Hospitals Coventry and Warwickshire, Sherwood Forest Hospitals, and Barking, Havering and Redbridge University Hospitals.

There are more crises to come. Monitor is building up a £300 million war chest, sufficient to send in special administrators to as many as sixty financially challenged trusts.[34] The Tories were happy in opposition to make political capital of challenging the way in which Tony Blair's Labour Government implemented the

Tory policy of PFI. And they are eager now to blame bad PFI deals on the previous government. Labour is still ignoring its own conference decisions and clinging stupidly to its discredited policy.

In office, of course, the Tories are the ones working most vigorously to prop up the PFI schemes and extend them, signing dozens of new ones for hospitals and other projects. It seems unlikely that the government will recognise the need for intervention, say, by pulling existing projects back into public ownership and thus stemming the flow of public money into private pockets. This is despite the fact that Monitor's chief executive David Bennett has suggested that it might be more advantageous to buy out the Peterborough PFI rather than have the NHS keep up the rising payments for thirty years.[35]

LIMITS TO PRIVATE INTEREST

Even while the public sector is cut back, the aftermath of the Francis Report has highlighted the limits to the private sector's ambitions to take over from the NHS. Many campaigners and commentators had expected the report's grim catalogue of revelations of failed services, callous and incompetent management, and stressed, short-handed staff delivering dangerously inadequate levels of care in Mid Staffordshire to be followed by a strident campaign by the *Daily Mail* and other rightward-leaning media for more services to be handed over to the private sector. But the campaign never happened. No one has suggested that the private sector is the solution to Mid Staffordshire.

Why? Because the services at the centre of the crisis, starved of resources and cut beyond any safe limit by desperate managers obsessed with financial targets, were precisely the services that the private sector does not provide. Things such as emergency care,

care for the chronic sick, health care for the elderly: all areas that private providers have branded as risky, complex and *unprofitable*. Nowhere in the world does the private sector voluntarily undertake this work – unless the company has been generously rewarded for accepting those risks as part of a lucrative contract. This is one reason why private hospitals are so small, averaging just fifty beds in England; in most cases, they do not have beds for emergencies, complex care, intensive therapy or similar care-intensive treatment. They are equipped and staffed to treat elective cases – most of them relatively prosperous, healthy individuals with private health insurance. Some beds are now being filled by cherry-picked NHS cases – picking up payments from the public purse so that no bed is left empty and unprofitable.

The private health sector that emerged in the last decade is an artificial creation, a product of favourable policies and government sponsorship. It continues to focus only on elective treatment, leaving the messy and complex work of caring for the poor and chronic sick to the NHS. And in the US, where the private sector delivers health care to the general population, the poor and those made poor by chronic illness, especially in old age, have been left to the government to care for, via the Medicaid programme – *because* they are not profitable patients. For this reason, the private sector could never be the solution to our country's health needs. The growth of the private sector can only be at the expense of the NHS, the very institution that boldly brought in care for all without charge, even in the depths of postwar austerity – the very institution that has proved beyond doubt that there are better alternatives to a competitive market in health care.

Ever since the postwar years, when Winston Churchill time and again led his party through the lobbies to oppose the formation of the NHS, the Conservative Party's mission has been to kill off the service that shares risk across the whole population, allocates resources according to health needs rather than market forces, and embodies the collective values and social solidarity Thatcher so openly despised when she insisted there was 'no such thing as society'. Now, sixty-five years later, David Cameron has revived some of the nastiest traditions of his party and enlisted the Liberal Democrats in his efforts to wind the clock back to a period many thought we had left behind.

Sadly, there is no sign so far of any equivalent courage or radicalism in the leadership of the Labour Party, which has vaguely promised to repeal the Health and Social Care Act 2012 but has taken no lead in reaching out to unite broader forces and build wider campaigns against it, and which further presents no clear conception of a viable path to undoing the damage that has been done to the NHS by Tory and Labour 'reforms' of the past decade. Indeed, Labour leaders seem trapped in a pointless battle to justify their party's mistaken and failed policies, rather than fighting the present threats and offering an alternative.

Aneurin Bevan famously argued that the NHS would live as long as there were people with the courage to defend it. The task today is to find those people and organise a rearguard fight, while there is still some trace of a recognisable NHS left for us to defend.

2

READY FOR MARKET

Stewart Player

*The state has to actively create a market, they don't
appear of their own account.*

Paul Corrigan,
former special health adviser to Tony Blair

In the many debates during the passage of Andrew Lansley's Health
and Social Care Bill, Coalition ministers repeatedly pointed out
that there was little substantial difference between the contents
of the bill and the policies of the previous government. Labour
health spokespeople squirmed but were unable to deny this charge
convincingly. In hindsight it is plain that New Labour's reforms
prepared the way for Lansley's drive to privatise the NHS, but it
wasn't so obvious at the time. A core group of policymakers largely
concealed their market-friendly intentions with rhetoric promoting
a re-envisioned 'GP-led', 'patient-centred' NHS based on 'choice'.
The terms 'contestability', 'increased local accountability' and
'world class' standards were in the mix as well.

Lansley's 'liberating' bill was the final step of a campaign, conceived as far back as the 1980s, by individuals closely linked to the private health industry. These visionaries imagined an England in which profits could once again be made through the delivery of health services. They were supported by key figures in Whitehall, not least in the Department of Health (DoH), where market-oriented thinking had become prevalent starting most especially in the Thatcher years. By the turn of the century advocates of instituting a health care market in Britain were increasingly pushing at an open door.

'MANAGED' CARE

In January 2002 the *British Medical Journal* (*BMJ*) published an article claiming that the giant California-based health care corporation Kaiser Permanente achieved higher levels of performance than the NHS at roughly the same cost.[1] Patients enrolled in the company's 'managed care plans' were said to experience 'more comprehensive and convenient primary care services and much more rapid access to specialist services and hospital admissions' than NHS patients. The article's authors also claimed that, by giving primary care physicians a tighter 'gatekeeper' function and emphasising management of chronic conditions, the corporation was able to limit the number of patients admitted to hospital, one of the more expensive aspects of health care.

Critics immediately pointed out that the article's statistics were hopelessly flawed – Kaiser's costs were higher than suggested and the NHS's patient base was on average older, and that in addition the article overlooked the multitude of functions – from medical education to public health – that the NHS performs but which Kaiser did not. Given that Kaiser's costs were roughly the same as those of the NHS, it was in reality far more expensive.[2]

The *BMJ* article helped to justify the extension of market principles into the NHS while reassuring everyone that Kaiser's 'not-for-profit' highly integrated system had a great deal in common with the NHS. Yet the *BMJ* authors were actually wrong about Kaiser's status too. In a letter to the *New England Journal of Medicine* a doctor at Kaiser pointed out that the physician group was directly linked to the Permanente Medical Group, a privately held, *for-profit* corporation, with a chief executive officer and a board of directors.[3] Yet the DoH's director of strategy, Chris Ham, defended the article's claims and Kaiser Permanente emerged as the model for NHS reform. DoH policymakers visited the company's headquarters in northern California and invited Kaiser staff to give seminars in London.

But behind the DoH's embrace of the Kaiser model stood a powerful economic fact. Throughout most of the 1990s, US managed care organisations (MCOs), and in particular the format known as health maintenance organisations (HMOs), had reaped huge profits and had become known as the 'Darlings of Wall Street'. The US government provided considerable support to MCOs in the belief that they would stimulate competition among health plans, increase efficiency and slow the growth in health care expenditures. Lower premiums also proved a considerable incentive for employers to adopt the schemes, and by the mid-1990s MCOs accounted for upwards of 90 per cent of the health care insurance cover in the US.

However, by 1998, these companies faced significant losses, owing to market saturation, government and employer strategies to contain health care costs, and high-profile scandals. To restore profitability, the US health care industry began to lower benefits to patients, increase premium fees and withdraw from selected domestic markets. Crucially, at this juncture a transition from national to multinational managed care began to take place. With the support of the World Bank and other US-led multilateral financial institutions, the industry now aimed to export 'managed care initiatives that convert public health care institutions and social insurance funds to private management, private owner-ship, or both' around the world.[4] Not only US but also European multinationals, including pharmaceutical companies and MCOs, began to seek markets abroad, and were particularly interested in the potential of state-funded health care systems. And, as Waitzkin has pointed out:

> Corporations exported managed care as the main organisational format, as opposed to other forms of commercial insurance, because managed care had become the dominant form of healthcare organi-sation in the US and had emerged as a profitable framework for commercial organisations to provide health insurance.[5]

The DoH's enthusiasm for the Kaiser model was therefore not simply an abstract fantasy but a response to a global shift towards health care privatisation, and to major influx of health care cor-porations from other countries interested in the NHS.

Kaiser is only one of several different models of commercially managed care in the US. All have the same goal: reducing costs and ensuring profits whilst maintaining quality of care. Before the advent of managed care, Americans mainly received their health services through employment-based insurance schemes, where a person could see any doctor or attend any hospital that had made arrangements to accept the insurance company's payouts for spe-cific care. This fee-for-service route was proving highly expensive, because doctors and hospitals stood to make more money if they ordered more tests and provided more treatments. Managed care sought to transform this by enabling commercial health care companies to take on the business of financing and insurance and in deciding how service provision would be organised and paid for. Premiums are negotiated between MCOs and both employers and state, as well as individuals, and generally a fixed premium includes all care services provided for in a contract. It is then up to these companies to provide such care packages while making a profit, which is largely achieved through contracts with selected networks of providers, as well as through rigorous control of hospital admissions, chronic disease management programmes and strict utilisation review. The providers themselves are paid by the MCO, primarily on a capitated, fixed-sum basis, and while the scale of the contracts is a strong incentive for these providers to become part of such networks, this form of payment puts a rein on indiscriminate delivery.

In organisational terms, managed care is essentially about the forms of relationship among MCOs (or insurers), and hospitals and physicians, and the extent of integration between these three parts.[6] For example, hospitals and physicians can come together into a physician hospital organisation (PHO), which is then well placed to win block contracts from MCOs or government programmes such as Medicare, which provides health care for Americans aged sixty-five or older. A group of doctors might instead decide to organise into an independent practitioner association (IPA), which can serve as both the provider of health care and an insurer for health care coverage, or can operate solely as a provider of services for patients enrolled in an MCO. Kaiser combines all three parts – insurance, hospitals and physicians – in a single integrated entity, where the insurer owns the hospitals and the physicians are salaried employees of the health plan.[7]

While the DoH was particularly interested in pursuing the Kaiser model, it remained open to other options for converting the NHS into a market. It was clear, however, that two changes were necessary before this could occur. First, the existing structures of the unified NHS had to be dissolved into the separate component parts of insurance and delivery. Second, these parts had to be reassembled into one or other of the managed care formats. Since any immediate proposal to introduce individual health insurance in place of the existing, tax-funded free service would be political suicide, the component of service delivery would be tackled first. In a favourite term used by DoH strategists, hospitals and physicians needed to be 'decoupled' from the NHS.

CUSTOMERS BEFORE PATIENTS

For hospitals such decoupling began in 2002 by making them into largely autonomous businesses called foundation trusts (FTs). These would be supervised not by the DoH but by an independent regulator, Monitor, and rather than offering a full range of health care services to their patients, FTs would receive a licence from Monitor to offer a specified number of services. The FTs were free to borrow on the private financial markets, enter into joint ventures with private companies and set their own terms of service for staff – a new level of financial and managerial freedom. The counterpart to these business freedoms was that the hospitals could no longer turn to the DoH if they ran up unsustainable debts. In other words they could go bust. In such a case Monitor would either step in, remove the management and invite another FT (or a private company) to take over, or simply let the hospital close. Financial viability became the overriding measure of a hospital's success, rather than whether it was serving the needs of the patients in its catchment area.

This was not the way that FTs were sold to Parliament and the public, however. Labour's Health Secretary, Alan Milburn, told the House of Commons that the bill introducing the new FT structure was built on three principles: 'community empowerment, staff involvement and democratisation'. 'In no way', he said, could the bill 'be reasonably described as privatisation, or a step in that direction'.[8]

The transformation of NHS hospitals into businesses was accelerated with the introduction in 2003 of a funding mechanism known as 'payment by results', whereby hospitals were paid per each individual who completed treatment, rather than with a lump sum for a given number of cases. Income now became closely tied to performance, which was measured by 'throughput', and payments were based on a national tariff of fixed prices, adjusted for the seriousness of each case category, not on how well patients did after they were treated. 'Payment by results' was actually a misleading name for the arrangement – it should have been 'payment by throughput'. It was another piece of policy bought wholesale from the US.

Another crucial, complementary step was the introduction of privately owned and operated independent sector treatment centres (ISTCs) to treat NHS patients, ostensibly in order to help tackle the backlog of patients waiting for standard, low-risk elective procedures such as cataract removals and knee and hip replacements. This step broke a long-standing taboo on allowing private companies to provide NHS clinical services, giving them access to significant amounts of NHS monies, attracting new companies from abroad to enter the market and enabling existing British ones to adapt their business structures to the new opportunities. The private health care industry began to transform itself from small-scale, expensive niche-market operators serving private patients to organisations capable of providing higher volumes of care at lower costs – the initial terms they were offered were highly favourable and virtually risk-free. These changes were reinforced by the formation inside the DoH of a Commercial Directorate, tasked with introducing private companies into the health service.[9]

ISTCs were modelled on American 'ambulatory care centres' (also sometimes alarmingly termed 'focused factories'), in which clinics handling elective procedures are separated from other surgical work, and composed of dedicated surgical teams. While ISTCs were supposed to provide their own staff, in practice NHS surgeons and support staff did most of the work, officially during their non-NHS working hours. This dependence on NHS staff made it clear that getting private providers to compete with NHS providers on a much larger scale would mean the permanent transfer of staff out of the NHS into either employment by private companies, or into companies or clinical networks (much like the American independent practitioner associations) that they would set up themselves.

NEXT TARGET: DOCTORS

This process was facilitated by new contracts made with hospital consultants in 2002, and with GPs in 2004. As far as DoH strategists were concerned, the bulk of the NHS workforce – its less formally skilled component – was seen as replaceable and could be transferred to private employers compulsorily; this had already happened on a large scale for cleaning, catering, laundry and portering staff, and would be extended to technical staff in outsourced diagnostic laboratories and other services. The situation was, however, very different for consultants and GPs. Creating the conditions under which they would also have to leave the NHS, or want to, was more of a challenge.

The government's approach to a new contract for consultants called for the imposition of productivity targets, tighter managerial control of workloads, and strict limits on the amount of private practice they could undertake. While these demands reflected a defensible concern to ensure that the highest-paid members of the workforce gave value for money, the government knew that they were anathema to most consultants, and cut to the heart of their professionalism and autonomy. As the then deputy chair of the BMA Consultants Committee, Jonathan Fielden, put it: the government had 'made fundamental errors in its understanding of the consultant contract and uses crude measures that focus on fast throughput instead of quality'.[10]

The clash over the consultants' contracts could be seen, and was generally seen, as the government trying to take on a privileged section of the workforce in the interests of patients and the taxpayer. But an article that appeared in the *Guardian* in November 2002, just after the consultants in England had angrily rejected the initial contract, put a very different complexion on the affair. It said that the rejection could 'have positive and far-reaching implications for the way NHS care is delivered – not least because it may open the door to more private sector provision of healthcare'.[11]

What was significant about this article is that it was written by Dr Penny Dash, who had been director of strategy at the DoH and a key architect of the 2000 NHS Plan when the new contract was conceived. The article revealed a rather different line of thinking inside the department. It spelled out the various ways in which consultants might escape control by NHS managers and suggested that in reality ministers might 'want to encourage surgeons, and indeed other groups of doctors, to form their own companies (or join existing private health providers) to sell their services back to the NHS'. 'Freed from the stifling grip of the NHS', Dash wrote, such companies could negotiate with the NHS to perform procedures in either NHS or private hospitals, or form businesses of their own, raising capital and investing in new technology, or joining up with suppliers of X-ray machines and scanners and offering a 'full service solution' to ailing NHS hospitals. Such a development, she suggested, could be what 'Messrs Blair and Milburn really wanted'.

Certainly the strategy had its desired effect. By August 2003 a survey found that the vast majority of consultants were considering a change of career, moving abroad or leaving the NHS to establish private 'chambers' (on the lines of barristers' chambers) through which they could sell their services to a variety of commissioning organisations, whether or not that involved the NHS. This last option was precisely what the government seemed to have been hoping for, according to Dr Dash. Only 23 per cent of the doctors surveyed said they were prepared to stay in the NHS till their retirement.[12]

The new GP contract operated rather differently, though in the context of a similar level of dissatisfaction among GPs at the time. On the surface, the new contract appeared to offer GPs everything they wanted, including significant pay rises and the ability to opt out of providing out-of-hours cover. Within a short time, over 90 per cent of GPs had opted out. But accepting these terms soon proved to be an own goal for doctors. It undermined the legitimacy they had previously enjoyed as the sole providers of primary care, and GPs very soon began to be pictured as an overpaid and outmoded profession, unwilling to respond to changing patient needs by opening their surgeries in the evenings and on Saturdays. This message was taken up and reiterated by the Commons Public Accounts Committee, the National Audit Office, the CBI and the media. From then on, few news stories about GPs would fail to mention their high pay and the question of weekend access.

Moreover, the scale of the opt-out from out-of-hours provision was something that the government fully anticipated and wanted. Out-of-hours provision also proved to be a useful entry point into primary care for private companies, an opening soon exploited on a growing scale by such companies as Serco and Harmoni. Another element in this process was a new Alternative Provider Medical Services (APMS) contract that allowed PCTs to commission primary care services from large private companies such as UnitedHealth Group, Care UK and Atos Origin, as well as from 'entrepreneurial' GP consortia and social enterprises, all of which employed GPs on a salary. All APMS contracts made provision for out-of-hours services and were targeted at 'under-doctored' areas, thereby further legitimising private sector provision.

These developments were followed, in 2007–08 by a new government initiative to move all GP practices in England into a system of 'polyclinics', also known variously as 'GP-led care centres', 'community health centres', 'walk-in centres' or 'Darzi centres' (so-named after the surgeon ennobled and made a government minister to front the idea). GPs therefore found themselves threatened with being forced to move into the new centres, while alternative commercial models of primary care were proposed in which the personalised patient care so valued by GPs would be replaced by Asda, Tesco or Virgin-based 'brands'. Payments to GP practices were also frozen at the 2004 level for three consecutive years, the government arguing that any increase would have to be linked to extended hours of access.

By 2010, 227 GP surgeries and health centres in England were being run by private companies, with nine firms (including Care UK and Assura Medical) each holding ten or more contracts. In March 2010 Virgin bought a majority stake in Assura and subsequently rebranded Assura's GP provider companies, or 'GPCos', as Virgin Care. Not all of these new commercial primary-care companies were small and, following the deal, Virgin Care claimed to administer twenty-five partnerships with over 1,500 GPs catering for over three million patients. However, in October 2012 some 300 of these GPs ended their partnership, owing to possible conflicts of interest with their new commissioning roles, and Virgin took full control over the GPCos.

POINTS OF ENTRY

The process of creating a market could naturally never be linear or tidy. The loosening of consultants' and GPs' ties to the NHS, for example, didn't occur simultaneously but in a seemingly disjointed series of policy developments, including contract adjustments and an ever-growing number of new entry points for private providers. By 2006 however, the policymakers felt confident that the component parts of managed care were sufficiently developed to begin to map out the next phase of transformation – i.e. assembling them into new market-based organisational formats. In that year a body called the National Leadership Network was formed, comprising 150 health policymakers, management consultants, NHS trust and private health care executives, as well as clinicians, professional leaders and regulators, to 'provide collective leadership for the next phase of transformation, advise ministers on developing policies and promote shared values and behaviours'.[13]

The National Leadership Network (NLN) soon produced a document entitled 'Strengthening local services: The future of the acute hospital',[14] which shows how the policymaking community was now envisaging myriad new forms of organisation and contractual relations between 'networked' organisations. For example, it thought that clinical staff would no longer be tied to working in particular settings, but would be available to work in whatever places were most appropriate. They would be organised in independent groups, such as multidisciplinary teams and 'managed clinical networks', and provide their services on a contractual basis to both NHS and other providers. 'Large chronic disease management companies' might consider joint ventures with 'clusters of GP commissioners', or possibly commissioners could allocate resources for specific care pathways to a 'principal provider', which could either provide such a package of care itself or subcontract elements of this package to other providers.

The NLN strategists clearly had in view the creation of an English version of 'managed care', and the range of organisational relationships that are typical of that system. Also belonging to this framework was the emphasis on dealing with chronic care and keeping hospital admissions to a minimum and with different forms of integration between hospitals, primary care providers, out-of-hours services, and social and domiciliary care providers and networks.

One early attempt to realise something of this approach was seen in the 'polyclinics' programme. Not only would this involve a radical redistribution of work away from hospitals, and the relocation to the polyclinics of most GPs and many hospital consultants, but also these new 'supersurgeries' would, like most new NHS hospitals, be privately financed, and quite likely privately owned and even operated. In October 2007 dispensing with any consultation, the DoH announced that it was providing £250 million to support the development of 152 polyclinics, one for each primary care trust (PCT) in England. The debt crisis of 2008, however, largely put paid to the programme. Although 140 polyclinics were established, in one form or another – of which over one-third were run by private companies or joint ventures with private companies – few, if any, resembled the bustling, high-tech, multipurpose facilities foreshadowed by the DoH and many were closed eventually. It is a fair bet, however, that similar institutions will resurface if the post-Lansley market evolves as intended.

Despite this setback, significant inroads were being made in transforming service delivery. It was always anticipated that the ISTC programme would serve as a precursor for a much wider range of clinical activity to be procured from private hospital providers. With the new business models put in place by local companies under the stimulus of the ISTC programme, private hospital chains such as Nuffield, BMI, Spire and Ramsay were now far better placed to pursue and expand their returns from NHS work. As Paul Corrigan, one of Labour's special health care advisers put it: 'the idea behind ISTCs was always something much bigger. We were always looking beyond the capacity hump. We never saw it as one big push and then waving goodbye to the private sector.'[15]

By 2011 private hospitals and clinics were doing almost £1 billion worth of NHS treatments. And by 2010 the deficit problems of many NHS trusts were also providing an entry point for such companies to take over NHS hospitals. One solution to the problem of trusts being unable to pass the financial survivability tests allowing them to become foundation trusts was that they could be either merged with an existing FT, or be taken over by private companies in franchise deals. In 2011 some sixty NHS hospitals run by twenty trusts were said to be in serious financial trouble and facing possible takeover, potentially by a private sector company such as Circle, which is already running Hinchingbrooke NHS hospital in Cambridgeshire. In June 2012 Candace Imison, deputy policy director of The King's Fund and a prominent

member of the National Leadership Network, said in a King's
Fund 'breakfast seminar' that 'evidence from McKinsey, using
international examples, suggests that takeovers by hospital chains
might be among the most successful approaches, particularly if
they reconfigure services'.[16] One can only assume that McKinsey
and Imison had the hospital chains of Spire, Ramsay, BMI and
others in mind.[17]

In October 2012 the House of Commons Public Accounts
Committee reported that one in five NHS trusts were in serious
financial difficulties, and that there was 'a real concern that some
would fail'.[18] The report came as administrators appointed to
oversee the crisis-hit South London Healthcare NHS Trust recommended that it be broken up and run by neighbouring NHS
trusts, or offered to private companies. Thirty-nine organisations
expressed interest in running parts of the trust, including Circle,
Care UK, Serco and Virgin Care.[19]

A considerable number of more entrepreneurially minded
GPs began to form their own private companies. While many
of these were modest affairs, by 2010 the trend was already
towards amalgamation and a search for wider geographical reach.
For example, in November 2010 one of the early market leaders, Chilvers McCrea, was bought by The Practice plc, which
itself held a range of public sector contracts, including twenty-
three NHS Local Improvement Finance Trust (LIFT) schemes,
six GP walk-in centres and seven contracts for prison health
services. Perhaps to fit in with NLN's vision of provider networks, the new combined company initially called itself Practice
Networks, and with large private equity backing it was able to
boast in 2013 that it had 'contracts for over 50 GP surgeries
and GP-led Health Centres, regularly delivers over 120 community outpatient clinics per week, and sees in excess of one
million patients per year'.[20]

BRINGING BACK INSURANCE

Getting rid of the whole idea of paying for people's health care out of general taxation, and restoring the principle of people paying individually for health insurance (with some government help for those too poor to pay for insurance), has long been the aim of the far Right. But actually shifting to it is fraught with political danger, so this final, and indeed critical, part of the American managed care model has been approached with extreme caution. The most obvious way to begin introducing private insurers into the NHS was through commissioning.

Under Labour this was to be achieved through a Framework for Procuring External Support for Commissioners (FESC), and a programme called World Class Commissioning. The idea was that major health care insurers from both the US and UK, as well as global consultancy companies with health care divisions, would be centrally involved in decisions by PCTs as to where, when, how and by whom services would be provided.[21] Service planning and 'reconfiguration' (which in this context all too often means cutting services) and the control of referrals, as well as explicitly market-oriented tasks such as marketing, would be increasingly farmed out to companies such as UnitedHealth, McKinsey, Aetna and BUPA.[22]

The incoming Coalition Government's decision to shift commissioning from PCTs to GPs organised in clinical commissioning groups was driven by a variety of motives, not least the growing impatience of the FESC companies with the level of business they actually got from the programme. Joint ventures were few and far between and small-scale, and there was resistance to outsourcing all commissioning work to the FESC companies, partly because of the continuing allegiance of many senior PCT staff to the public service concept of the NHS. GPs were seen as more pliable, whether because of a latent entrepreneurialism among an influential minority, or because of their 'independent contractor' relationship to the NHS, or simply because they had enough on their hands taking care of patients and so would be ready to hand over effective control of commissioning (and hence control of the bulk of the NHS budget) to private companies.

In practice, long before the Health and Social Care Act 2012 had completed its parliamentary passage, the government was already assigning far bigger commissioning roles to private companies. In October 2011, for example, NHS London announced that thirty-one out of thirty-eight of the capital's clinical commissioning groups (CCGs) were to sign contracts with private firms for a programme of 'intensive organisational support' for a range of activities including governance, organisational development and strategy, finance, market analysis, leadership plans, resources, how-to guides, and self-assessment tools – which, it has to be said, covers pretty much everything.[23] They also took responsibility for QIPP (quality, innovation, productivity and prevention) – a quintessential example of management consultant phrasing. After the passage of the act, these arrangements were to be formalised in the shape of commissioning support organisations, which would compete with each other to do the commissioning on behalf of CCGs.

The installation of private health insurers at the heart of NHS commissioning seems bound to advance the time when private insurance begins to complement, if not displace, public funding for NHS care. If patients are encouraged to take out insurance to 'top up' an increasingly narrowing range of free services, or services of declining quality, insurance 'products' or packages custom-made for the purpose will be ready and available, designed by insurers close to the scene of action. PCTs are already restricting access to some treatments, such as cataract removals, hernia operations, and hip and knee replacements, by raising the threshold of how ill or disabled a patient has to be, with a corresponding rise in self-pay products offered by insurers.

Another route to private insurance that seems likely to expand is personal care budgets, which are being rolled out for NHS patients with complex ongoing conditions. Like all budgets, these are likely to prove finite, with the invitation to 'top them up' for needs that the budgets won't cover, but which can be insured for. These were initially piloted in June 2009 with provisional status awarded to sixty-eight personal-health-budget projects in seventy-five PCTs, but even before this the private health insurance sector was anticipating their impact and preparing new products to cover the top-ups for which a demand could sooner or later be expected.[24] In March 2009 AXA PPP's commercial director said: 'We welcome the DH's decision to allow patients to complement their NHS treatment with privately funded care. It's a big step in the right direction of giving patients greater choice over their healthcare provision.'[25] The Coalition Government has made it clear that personal budgets should be offered to other patients in due course.

PUTTING IT ALL TOGETHER

While Labour constructed the building blocks of managed care, assembling them into a coherent whole has certainly accelerated under the Coalition Government. The linked 'policy community' of think tanks and management consultancies has been increasingly emboldened to propose a range of possible formats, including integrated care organisations (ICOs), local clinical partnerships, GP federations, the Circle model and accountable lead organisations. All have direct counterparts in the US system. The leading think tanks, The King's Fund and Nuffield Trust in particular, have advocated all of these formats, drawing on seminars with executives from US organisations such as Geisinger, Hill Physicians, Ford Health Systems and of course Kaiser. The content of such meetings often concerns 'clinical leadership' within such organisations, though 'mentoring doctors for the market' would be a more accurate description of what they have to offer. In England, the channels for this have been growing: the National Association for Primary Care is linked with UnitedHealth; the Royal College of General Practitioners, with McKinsey (and previously with Aetna); and the NHS Alliance opened a commissioning college with Humana.

The GP federations and integrated care organisations (ICOs) deserve a closer look. The federation model of physician groupings was developed between 2007 and 2011 under the aegis of the Royal College of General Practitioners (RCGP) during the chairmanship of Professor Steve Field. In the college's original 'roadmap', produced in 2007, federations were described as 'group[s] of practices and primary care teams working together, sharing responsibility for developing high quality, patient focused services for their local communities'.[26] The future of GP federations is fairly unclear, particularly in terms of whether they should adopt both commissioning and service delivery functions, or simply act as providers of care, but they are still under active consideration. Federations can indeed act as commissioning consortia, and at least six were chosen in the first two waves of clinical commissioning pathfinders. Through the assumption of financial and performance risk, and adoption of economies of scale, there is the possibility that these can act in the same way as American IPAs, which contract with insurance plans to manage the care of patients within a fixed annual budget.[27]

But a 'toolkit', produced in 2010 jointly by the RCGP, The King's Fund and the Nuffield Trust, put more flesh on the federation model, suggesting various formats, ranging from private companies limited by shares or guarantees to community interest companies and limited liability partnerships. When the toolkit was produced, 15 per cent of federations were already working with an external partner, including Virgin Assura and Aetna. The Leeds-based Leodis organisation, for example, comprises a commissioning arm; 121 member GPs from 27 practices; and, with public and private partners, including Barclays Private Equity, a joint venture company whose 'mission' is to 'build enhanced health care centres and clinics for general practices, locally based diagnostic and outpatient services'. Despite this, the RCGP toolkit favoured separating commissioning from the provision of care; a federation, the RCGP maintained, should be a 'provider entity that can tender for services offered by a future GP commissioning consortium'.

The integrated care organisation model might better fulfil the yearnings of The King's Fund and Nuffield Trust crowd. The aim of integration is widely supported – on the assumption that it means reducing fragmentation of patient services and enabling better co-ordinated care.[28] It remained for the influential pro-market Policy Exchange think tank, in a report published in November 2012, to make clear what 'integrated care' actually means to leading policymakers.[29] It called for a pilot programme of ten full-scale NHS ICOs, each covering a population of around 250,000, bringing together primary, community and acute services into one organisation with a single budget for the purchase and provision of services. The report thought the impetus for the model would come from the financial failure of some NHS hospital trusts, which would make ICOs a palatable alternative to service closure. It envisaged GPs being offered £160,000 each for the goodwill of their practices and becoming salaried employees, and thought that private sector management 'should not be controversial in principle'. Monitor officials have also suggested that the organisations should house a range of private providers offering, for example, diabetes care and orthopaedics, and all 'sharing their excellence'.[30]

The Policy Exchange's model is a close equivalent of the Kaiser organisation, only with (it assumed) continued funding from taxes rather than private health insurance. Just weeks after the publication of the report, however, the chair of Monitor, Dr David Bennett, announced that private companies could become the 'lead' contractors to commission services on behalf of clinical commissioning groups, and no doubt this option will be extended to ICOs if the Policy Exchange's proposal is taken up. The idea is very much alive in policymaking circles. Shortly after the publication of his book, *Never Again?*, on the passage of the health bill, Nicholas Timmins, the former *Financial Times* health correspondent and part-time fellow at The King's Fund, foresaw 'patients choosing between competing integrated care organizations; a choice, so to speak, between a set of NHS Kaiser Permanentes'.[31]

LAST INCENTIVES

A recent paper has argued that the drive by US and multinational corporations from the end of the 1990s onwards to export managed care proved largely unsuccessful in Europe, with the popularity of public sector health care acting as 'a powerful disincentive to privatization', and that 'countries such as the UK, the Netherlands and Sweden reversed some (but not all) policies that attempted to privatize their national health programmes'. Although debates continued in recent years about both privatisation and marketisation, these 'did not lead to basic changes in the systems' fundamentally public character'. Instead US-based MCOs turned to less developed countries, in Latin America in particular, which, the authors continue:

> [E]xperienced strong pressure to accept managed care as the organisational framework for the privatization of their health systems. MCOs and investment funds rapidly entered the Latin American market, and this experience served as a model for the export of managed care to Africa and Asia.[32]

As far as the UK, or more accurately England, is concerned, we can only argue that the authors are mistaken. The processes involved have just been more covert. The seemingly disjointed series of policy developments, such as the formation of foundation trusts, new consultant and GP contracts, and the centrality of the commissioning function, as well as the ways in which these have been presented as being about increased efficiency, greater choice, a more plural range of providers, and increased local accountability, simply masked a largely coherent long-term strategy.

This strategy was, and continues to be, steadily pursued by the policy community both inside and outside the NHS, with no discernible difference of approach between the public and private sectors. Each step towards market formation has been consolidated by the formation of a new institution. Inside the NHS, for example, a Foundation Trust Network was formed in 2004, and an NHS Partners Network for private companies doing NHS work soon joined it. And outside – though not very far away, in practice – there was a group of well-funded think tanks, above all The King's Fund and the Nuffield Trust, which have been consistent, though seemingly cautious, advocates of managed care models. And then there is a wide range of interest groups, such as the PPP Forum, set up in 2001, 'the industry body for public private partnerships delivering UK infrastructure' (the largest part of which is for the NHS). One can also add the large, often global, management consultancies such as KPMG, PwC and Ernst & Young, whose staff have occupied, and often still occupy, pivotal positions within the DoH.

But in promoting the import of the US managed care framework, the most influential outside organisation by far has been the US consultancy giant McKinsey, whose clients include at least ninety of the Fortune 100 corporations. McKinsey's hand in drafting the health bill is now widely acknowledged, and the scale and range of the company's penetration of the corridors of governmental power in the interests of these clients is impossible to ignore. Following Dr Penny Dash's spell as head of strategy in the DoH, she became a McKinsey partner and played the leading role in producing Labour's two 'Darzi' reports, the first of which sought to radically restrict levels of provision and staffing in London, while the second envisaged the privately run polyclinic system. In 2004 Dash became a non-executive director of Monitor and also set up the Cambridge Health Network, a McKinsey front that brings together DoH policymakers with private company officials at meetings sponsored by some of the biggest names in US capital, from Halliburton to General Electric – hardly household names in health care, but all with a shared interest in replacing public services by private enterprise.

While David Bennett and two other former McKinsey partners occupy the leading positions in Monitor, the company's influence extends into many other key parts of the policy community. Dash is vice chair of The King's Fund, while another McKinsey partner, Nicolaus Henke, is vice chair of the second biggest health-policy think tank, the Nuffield Trust. Following the publication of the Policy Exchange report on ICOs, Bennett has shown considerable urgency in pushing the programme through; and ministers have shown themselves keen to avoid any unnecessary piloting and evaluation. Indeed at a recent meeting at The King's Fund with Monitor and the NHS Commissioning Board, the consensus was that the programme be 'allowed to suspend rules that got in the way of progress'. In January 2013 the *Health Service Journal* reported that while the programme might not progress quite as quickly as anticipated it had a strong supporter in David Cameron's chief policy adviser, Paul Bate – yet another former McKinsey staffer.

Everything looks to be in place for the increasing domination of the market over the NHS. The preparations have largely been hidden from view, and for good reason – there is not, and never has been, a political mandate for this momentous change, and certainly not for importing the US model of health care. And worse, the market mentality is ready to destroy the very public service ethos that has made the NHS so effective over the past sixty-five years.

3

PARLIAMENTARY BOMBSHELL

David Wrigley

Improving the NHS is the Conservative party's number one priority … this requires an end to the pointless upheavals, politically motivated cuts, increased bureaucracy and greater centralisation that have taken place under Labour.

David Cameron and Andrew Lansley, *NHS Autonomy and Accountability*

On 12 July 2010 Andrew Lansley landed his bombshell White Paper, 'Equity and excellence: Liberating the NHS', on Parliament. It signified the biggest assault on the NHS in its history, with collateral damage extending throughout the 1.7 million people working in the service and the sixty million citizens who depended on it. Two months earlier the Coalition had been forged, when David Cameron had failed to deliver an overall majority to his disappointed party, and made a deal with Nick Clegg in order to form the government. In the published Coalition agreement, a promise had been made to the electorate: 'We will stop the top-down reorganisations of the NHS that have got in the way of patient care.'

The events leading up to the public launch of Lansley's White Paper were noteworthy, to say the least. His plans for the NHS, which anticipated five years' worth of legislated changes, had been very well developed by the time of the general election, but they suddenly needed to be adapted, at short notice, to take account of the newly formed Coalition with the Lib Dems. The early discussions between the top ministers from the two parties hardly touched upon health, which few thought would be a contentious area. For instance, Nick Timmins, in his short book for The King's Fund, *Never Again?*, quotes a senior Liberal Democrat as saying: 'We [the Coalition] didn't have any other discussions about the NHS of any kind during those few days. We didn't discuss reform. I think if I'm honest the assumption probably was that the NHS was going to be an area where a degree of stability would be expected. NHS reform hadn't been one of our lead areas.'[1]

The job of producing a more detailed 'programme for government' for the Coalition agreement was given to Oliver Letwin, who, before the election, had been Conservative Shadow Chancellor of the Exchequer and had predicted publicly that the NHS would not exist five years after the Tories got back into power. In 1988 he had co-authored *Britain's Biggest Enterprise: Ideas for Radical Reform of the NHS* for the Right-leaning Centre for Policy Studies think tank. He was joined in the Coalition project from the Lib Dem side by Daniel 'Danny' Alexander MP, soon to become Chief Secretary of the Treasury. Lansley was sidelined while Letwin and Alexander slugged it out, trying to reconcile two fundamentally different approaches.

Health 'proved one of the more difficult areas'. Neither Letwin nor Alexander had any expertise in health policy, nor were special advisers with relevant experience assigned to the topic. The result was a compromise that may have pleased the protagonists but looked like an unworkable mess to anyone who understood health policy. Lansley later said, 'I did have conversations with Oliver Letwin from time to time, but to say they covered every aspect ...' showing that he felt sidelined.

In any case, when the language was finalised and the programme published on 20 May 2010, Lansley 'didn't like it'. Now officially Secretary of State for Health, he set out to work on a fudge with his department. Eventually, by envisioning a number of bold moves – including abolition of the primary care trusts (PCTs) and strategic health authorities (SHAs) in England – they came up with what Lansley felt was a workable plan – the plan presented in the White Paper for the first time that July day.

The White Paper provoked much surprise when it landed in Parliament, though perhaps it should not have. On 27 February 2010, at the Tories' spring conference, Lansley had given a keynote speech to rally the troops. He promised his audience that he would put a stop to the 'endless, pointless bureaucracy, costing the NHS billions extra every year'. Still, the idea of abolishing the PCTs and SHAs had not been mooted in any pre- or post-election talks or policy papers.

NHS staff were already 'reconfiguration weary', and this would entail yet more upheaval, yet more time and energy spent on a process of change to NHS structure rather than to patient care. Lansley may have taken aim at 'pointless' bureaucracy and billions in taxpayer's money, but analysts would subsequently calculate the cost of his reforms to be around £1.6 billion. As Professor Chris Ham wrote in the *BMJ*: 'A reorganisation that promised to reduce bureaucracy and streamline structures ... achieved exactly the opposite with consequences yet to be fully understood.'[2]

CONSULTING THE COUNTRY

During the following summer and autumn, numerous organisations and individuals set about digesting the White Paper and its supporting documents. This was the 'consultation' period to air out the suggestions put forward by Lansley and the Department of Health. The initial wave of responses varied widely.

Despite the radical nature of the plans, some welcomed a new approach to delivering healthcare. Yes, there was reason for concern over such a large reorganisation, as well as whether GPs were up to the challenge of controlling the commissioning of health care. Doctors would, in effect, through the clinical commissioning groups (CCGs) and the NHS Commissioning Board (NHSCB), be handed a £70 billion budget. The private sector, in particular, saw distinct possibilities for an expanded role in health care. Julia Manning is a former Conservative parliamentary candidate and chief executive of 2020health.org, a not-for-profit organisation that researches better health practices. She said: 'We see real opportunities as a result for private contractors and Social Enterprises to become much more involved in providing and facilitating NHS services.' Others voiced more caution, and acknowledged the ambition of the White Paper reforms. In a *BMJ* editorial, Chris Ham, chief executive of The King's Fund, remarked, 'Lansley came into office as a man with a plan.' Ham added, 'backing general practitioners … is both radical and risky'.

The British Medical Association's (BMA) response was still more muted. Its council chairman, Dr Hamish Meldrum, wrote to the medical profession on 30 July 2010: 'The BMA believes that it is absolutely vital that we critically engage with the consultation process. Government has clearly indicated its overall direction of travel and non-engagement in the consultation period would greatly increase the risk of bringing about the adverse outcomes that many of you fear.'[3] Most doctors understood why the BMA wished to engage with the consultation process but little did they know that this 'engagement' would continue well past the consultation period.

The BMA's GP Committee accepted the main thrust of the White Paper, despite significant opposition to its contents among the nation's GPs. *GP* magazine had conducted an initial survey on the White Paper and two-thirds of respondents opposed the plans to force practices to join commissioning consortia. One of the committee's senior members, Dr Beth McCarron-Nash, urged GPs to keep an open mind: 'There is more detail to come. What we end up with could be very different from what we are reading now.'[4] She was right, but not in the way she would have wished.

Over six thousand responses were sent in, from organisations ranging from 2020health.org to the YWCA.[5] A small number of responders saw Lansley's plans as an attempt to 'commercialise' the NHS, a project that, as we have seen, had started decades earlier in various guises. Unite, the UK's largest trade union, called the White Paper an 'untested, expensive exercise in political dogma'. Labour's Shadow Secretary of State for Health Andy Burnham declared that the reforms outlined in the White Paper would 'unpick the very fabric of the NHS'. According to the Socialist Health Association: 'The Coalition have not learned the lesson which it took Labour ten years to learn – that reorganisation is a diversion not a solution.' Yet, most of the initial responses during the consultation period were mainly concerned about the huge upheaval for the NHS, and the strain that would be put on doctors taking on the responsibility for health care commissioning. Less notice was taken of the future role that might emerge for commercial health care providers.

Later, once the dust had settled, Chris Ham would call this out as one of the decisive points in the process: 'Although many organisations ... focused their attention on plans to give general practices a major role in commissioning ... these changes are of secondary importance compared with the radical extension of competition.'[6]

NEXT STEPS

On 15 December 2010 the Department of Health published 'Liberating the NHS: Legislative framework and next steps',[7] which outlined the government's response to the consultation submissions. A series of fact sheets were also issued, covering 'economic regulation', 'local democratic legitimacy' and 'commissioning for patients' – the latter of which noted: 'Key decisions affecting patient care should be made by healthcare professionals in partnership with patients and the wider public, rather than by managerial organisations.' Little attention had been paid to the many and legitimate concerns that had been raised during the consultation; instead, there was lip service. It quickly became clear that Lansley was not in listening mode, and that storm clouds were gathering.

Some proposals rang alarm bells. Most of the press focus was on the decision to put maternity commissioning under the control of local GP commissioners and not the national NHS Commissioning Board as originally planned. Lansley remained confident about his chances for passage and stated 'our reform agenda is on track'.

The next month, on 19 January 2011, Lansley's Health and Social Care Bill was presented to Parliament. It ran to 354 pages and 281 sections.[8] It was littered with elements that had not been in the manifestos of either party in the Coalition Government before the general election. One might easily come to the same conclusion as Michael Portillo: the Tories deliberately hid their NHS proposals from the public. 'They did not believe they could win an election if they told you what they were going to do because people are so wedded to the NHS', as Portillo told Andrew Neil.

The enormity and complexity of the proposed legislation caused considerable disquiet and it was very hard to understand what the bill would actually mean for practising doctors and their patients. Its contents demanded close and informed scrutiny, in particular around the role of the Secretary of State to provide health care and the effect it would have on how EU law applied in future, notably in relation to competition. Unfortunately, large organisations such as the British Medical Association, the Trades Union Congress and the Royal College of Nursing, with significant legal resources behind them, never undertook a full forensic analysis of the whole bill – something that could have shown from the outset how damaging it would be to the fabric of the NHS.

Much of this work was done by individuals, foremost among them Professor Allyson Pollock, public health physician and professor of public health research and policy at Queen Mary, University of London, and Peter Roderick, a public interest lawyer. Their work provided much of the information needed for parliamentarians and others to expose the true meaning behind the complex legal language in the bill. Further analysis of the legal implications was carried out by the online community group 38 Degrees. If other groups had supported them in exposing the reality behind the bland assurances, Lansley's plans might well have stalled.

As mentioned in the introduction, in January 2011 the independent and highly respected *BMJ* wrote a damning editorial entitled 'Dr Lansley's Monster', which was accompanied by an illustration of Frankenstein on the front cover.[9] The *BMJ* called the government 'mad' to be embarking on such changes and challenged their democratic legitimacy.

Early in the journey towards legislation, one Tory MP spoke out repeatedly, criticising the bill: Dr Sarah Wollaston, a GP who became Conservative MP for Totnes in 2010. She remarked that the Lansley bill was like 'tossing a hand grenade' into local health structures. In March 2011 she said: 'These proposals mean the NHS would go belly up, not top down', and claimed that key elements of the reorganisation were 'completely unrealistic and doomed to fail'. She went on: 'It is no use liberating the NHS from top down political control only to shackle it to an unelected economic regulator … There is a risk that commissioning consortia [are] "doomed to fail" and will hand over their commissioning to the private sector.'

Wollaston, who sits on the Health Select Committee, said she would have liked to have sat on the committee examining the government's health proposals in detail. But, she explained: 'When I suggested to the whips that I would like to table amendments, I effectively signed myself off the list of candidates. The intention appears to be to get the bill through committee unscathed with no amendments, unless suggested by the government.' She was unwilling to 'turn up on time, say nothing and vote with the government', as previously instructed by a party whip.

Later, Wollaston claimed that many of her concerns had been addressed after Lansley's bill was 'paused' and recommendations by the Future Forum were accepted into the draft legislation. It is difficult to avoid the conclusion that pressure had been brought to bear on her. At any rate, near the end of 2011 Wollaston was making helpful comments in support of the legislation, such as, 'it is better to focus on where we go from here rather than how we could have arrived by a less contentious route'; and, 'This is not the privatisation of the NHS.' She had less to say in the final, and more crucial, six months of the Health and Social Care Act's passage through Parliament. In 2012 she was one of the votes that made the bill law.

At an early stage the DoH asked local GPs working in fledgling commissioning groups to apply for what the department called 'pathfinder status' – an indication that they were getting ready to work as a full-blown CCG – in order to demonstrate that the bill had clinical 'buy in'. The intention was that this status would also show that these GPs would receive extra support from the NHSCB. In reality, such support never materialised to any great extent, and these pathfinder groups were used primarily as a demonstration that doctors supported the bill. Nothing could have been further from the truth, but the DoH's and the politicians' spin machine was put into motion, with Lansley and Cameron repeatedly mentioning these pathfinder groups in their speeches as justification of their claim that the legislation had clinical 'buy in'.

THE POLITICAL SHIELD

The Liberal Democrats had previously acted as the Tories' 'human shield' when pushing through policies that were unpopular with the electorate. They were to play a similar role during the debates over Lansley's bill, indeed proving absolutely vital to its passage through both houses of Parliament.

In early 2011, however, some members of the Liberal Democrat Party started to become concerned about the ramifications of Lansley's White Paper. (For more on this, see Charles West's chapter in this book.) They were unhappy that there had been no mention of the huge reorganisation involved, either in the election manifestos of the Coalition parties or, more importantly, in the post-election Coalition agreement. These concerned parties could point to the fact that the White Paper had been thrust upon a largely unsuspecting Westminster, a shocked NHS and a bemused public.

Foremost among them were Evan Harris, a doctor and former Lib Dem MP for Oxford West and Abingdon, and Baroness Shirley Williams, Lib Dem member of the House of Lords. Williams summed up her feelings thus: 'I had an instinct if you like. I just felt very deeply that this was something that was completely misconceived.'[10] She went on to call Lansley's bill an act of 'stealth privatisation', stating: 'I can't support the coalition plan for the NHS. Why we should dismember this remarkably successful public service for an untried and disruptive re-organisation amazes me.'[11] Over the coming year, Williams's views on the Health and Social Care Bill would change dramatically, however, and with significant implications.

Harris for his part espoused a hopeful view of the Lib Dems' influence, stating in 2011 that: 'for the government as a whole and the Conservative party in particular, the biggest problem they face is the opposition of the Liberal Democrats to significant parts of the changes, expressed in very clear terms overwhelmingly at our party conference in Sheffield on 12 March'.[12]

At the Lib Dem spring party conference in 2011, several prominent members expressed unease, causing some panic in Whitehall. The Tories knew they needed the Lib Dems on side in order to achieve the arithmetical majority in the Commons when Lansley's bill went to vote. Something had to be done to try and assuage the concerns of their Coalition partners. The bill was in trouble.

Senior Lib Dems threatened that unless changes were made the bill would not get through the Lords. Lib Dem peers might feel more obliged to heed the concerns of the grass roots, and independent peers could not be whipped into line. The bill was tottering dangerously, with Nicholas Timmins reporting that there was even talk of killing it off.[13]

Cameron stepped in. During a discussion in the Cabinet room between Cameron and Nick Clegg, much seems to have been ironed out. 'Andrew Lansley is now increasingly sidelined,' said one Whitehall source, 'you have now got David Cameron listening to David Nicholson, so Andrew Lansley is less relevant.'

Clegg rejected the idea of killing off the bill, claiming it would be worse for the NHS to abandon it altogether than to proceed with an amended bill. In addition, Lansley had set moves in place to enact the changes before the legislation was passed, so that existing structures were already being broken up, and many people had left jobs. It made little difference now that Lansley wasn't centre stage, but things could still derail.

The leaders of the Coalition knew a potential political disaster when they saw one. Their answer was to call for a 'pause', and to inform Lansley to get on with it.

THE POLITICS OF 'PAUSE'

Consequently, on 4 April 2011 Secretary of State Andrew Lansley stood up in the House of Commons and made an announcement that surprised many: he would be 'pausing the bill' at a 'natural stage in its passage through Parliament'.[14] He continued: 'I can therefore tell the House that we propose to take the opportunity of a natural break in the passage of the Bill to pause, listen and engage with all those who want the NHS to succeed, and subsequently to bring forward amendments to improve the plans further in the normal way'.

At the time, many commented that there was nothing natural in pausing a bill as it passed through Parliament. But the pause went forward.

Lansley needed someone to head up the group – the Future Forum – who would 'listen' during this pause. He chose Professor Steve Field, former chair of the Royal College of General

Practitioners (RCGP), part-time GP in Birmingham and well-known supporter of the bill. The rest of the group comprised forty-four carefully hand-picked members.[15] A number of meetings were set up across England to 'engage' with the public and the profession. Online 'live debates' were held and there was much discussion in various forums.

While the private sector did not have direct representation at the Future Forum, they did not need to fear. Their interests were being well taken care of by others. Notable among the members of the Future Forum was Sir Stephen Bubb. As chief executive of the Association of Chief Executives of Voluntary Organisations, Bubb represented the views of not-for-profit providers of health care. He had already shown the direction of his recommendations in a blog promising 'radical proposals'. In May 2011 he wrote: 'I went to a good meeting today with the NHS Confed[eration] Partners Network, an umbrella body for all the independent providers in the health service. For political reasons, the private sector were excluded from the Future Forum, so in my area I feel it's only right to ensure I hear their views. And very balanced and sensible they are. I still hold to the view that what matters is what is delivered, not who delivers it.' Another member was David Worskett, head of the NHS Partners Network, whose members included the private health companies General Healthcare Group, Virgin Care, Harmoni Ltd, BUPA, Care UK and UnitedHealth UK.

When a member of the audience at one of the listening exercises asked 'How are private health companies' views being reflected on the Forum?' Worskett replied: 'The role of alternative providers is exactly the same for-profit and not-for-profit providers and we do have a number of absolutely wonderful not-for-profit providers represented on the Forum and, of course, Stephen Bubb, the chief executive of ACEVO is leading the competition work stream. I think I want to say publicly that I'm enormously grateful to him for the extraordinary competence and energy with which he is doing that.' Worskett went on to lament the fact that: 'The route [for the views of the private sector] is indirect [but] I don't think anybody needs worry with Stephen in full cry that the angles aren't being addressed.'

The *BMJ* also revealed lobbying by Worskett for his colleagues in the private health sector.[16] In a briefing paper published by the Social Investigations blog, Worskett wrote: 'Several members [of the NHS Partners Network] have used their own "routes" to gain access to key players within No 10 and have been able to report back that the stance there is supportive, though there is low awareness of exactly what the independent sector does or could do ... I did brief the new No 10 health policy adviser very fully, and indeed "cleared" our materials with him. I have had several other "stock-take" phone conversations with him. We are certainly on No 10's radar.' Worskett explained that DoH ministers and senior civil servants had given him 'every signal possible that they understood and sympathised with our concerns and shared our view of the key issues and priorities'. Assessing the tactics to be used during the remaining weeks of the pause, he added: 'We need to keep as close as possible to No 10 over the next few weeks ... As we move into the next phase we will need to shift our efforts onto the politicians – those the government listen to, and those who will play key roles in the House of Lords when the bill gets there.'

The same briefing paper, the *BMJ* said, also showed how individual members of the Future Forum were targeted so that the private sector would not be blocked from expanding its reach in the case that the Forum's final report to the Prime Minister recommended watering down the legislation. Again, quoting Worskett's own words: 'If the report by the NHS Future Forum to the Prime Minister went the wrong way for us, retrieving the position would be almost impossible ... Therefore the tactical imperative had to be to influence the Forum members directly and to concentrate other activity on those who themselves would have most influence on the Forum.' Worskett explained that he held 'lengthy' meetings with Stephen Bubb, who was serving as chairman of the Forum's working group on choice and competition. In those meetings, Worskett said: 'We agreed on the approach he would take, what the key issues are, and how to handle the politics.'

Some questioned Bubb's impartiality, notably John Pugh, the Lib Dem MP and spokesman for health, who commented: 'In particular, the role of Bubb in chairing the listening exercise on competition is seen by many as a clear conflict of interest. Asking Sir Stephen to sum up on competition rules is as neutral as asking Simon Cowell to tell us about the merits of TV talent shows.'

Quite how much listening took place during this period was unclear. At one Future Forum 'listening event', Bubb was heard to say in response to an awkward question on the role of competition in the NHS, 'I am not listening to that as I don't agree' – not quite the listening that many members of the public and NHS professionals might have been seeking. The response also flew in the face of Bubb's own comment on the DoH's website: 'So people can be assured when they're making comments to us we will listen to what they say.' It's no wonder that many who attended meetings, and those who weren't able to find one to attend, felt that the entire exercise was a sham.

While the listening sessions were mostly going to plan, there was some bad news for Lansley. On 13 April 2011 the Royal College of Nursing (RCN) annual conference met in Liverpool and in an unprecedented move voted 99 per cent in favour of a motion of 'no confidence' in Lansley's handling of the NHS reforms. The RCN are traditionally seen as more conservative than other nursing unions, so this was a major blow. The vote made numerous media headlines that day. In the aftermath, Lansley chose to meet with a small, hand-picked group of sixty RCN conference delegates when he visited the meeting after the vote. To the amazement of many in attendance, he apologised for not having got his message about the reforms across well enough to gain their support.

Then on 10 May 2011 he found some relief. A group of forty-five 'CCG GPs' wrote a letter to the *Telegraph* expressing their 'wholehearted support for the Coalition's health reforms'.[17] The letter, which had been orchestrated by Dr Jonathan Munday, a GP in Westminster and chair of the Victoria Commissioning Consortium, was used repeatedly by Lansley to demonstrate that there was support for the bill. Munday was a former Conservative councillor and mayor of Kensington and Chelsea. After criticisms began to pour in about the supportive nature of the letter, he said he was no longer a member of the Conservative Party and had 'nothing to do with Tory Central Office'.

Despite this show of support, Lansley could not keep the alarm bells from ringing. Around this time it emerged that a senior adviser to Cameron had made some unguarded comments a few months earlier to a conference in New York City. Mark Britnell, a former director of commissioning at the DoH, had begun working for KPMG, a management consultancy that had already made millions from advising the NHS and was set to make much more if Lansley's bill was enacted by Parliament. At the New York meeting, Britnell had reportedly said: 'GPs will have to aggregate purchasing power and there will be a big opportunity for those companies that can facilitate this process … In future, the NHS will be a state insurance provider, not a state deliverer.' He then added: 'The NHS will be shown no mercy and the best time to take advantage of this will be in the next couple of years.' Later, in an article for the *Health Services Journal*, he suggested that providing treatment entirely 'free at the point of care' was not necessary to the health service, and that 'top-up payments' would be beneficial to the NHS's own health. 'It appears that countries that have a mixed blend of public and private provision, co-payment and social insurance are possibly more capable of providing resilient healthcare systems', Britnell wrote. He provided no evidence for his assertion, however. In a response to the article, Dr Jonathon Tomlinson, a London GP and long-time campaigner for the NHS, said: 'This is hardly surprising, and a salutary warning about the ideology guiding NHS reforms.'

On 13 May 2011, just prior to filing the Future Forum final report with Cameron, Clegg and Lansley, Steve Field mentioned in an interview with the *Guardian* that the report would suggest that Monitor's primary duty – to enforce competition between health care providers – should be scrapped. Instead, he said Monitor should be obliged to do the opposite, by promoting co-operation and collaboration and the integration of health services.

THE FINAL FORUM

The Future Forum report, published on 13 June 2011, made sixteen key recommendations. Most of these were seen as a sop to the Lib Dems, designed to procure support for Lansley's ailing bill and to allow it to proceed on its parliamentary journey. The suggestions still kept the focus on the need for 'choice and competition', but this was downplayed by saying that competition would centre not on price but on *quality*. Many were able to read between the lines to understand that this would pave the way for the private sector to have a much bigger say in bidding for NHS contracts. 'Any Qualified Provider' status would remain in place. More controversially, the duties of the Secretary of State with respect to the NHS would be amended, though the government insisted that the Secretary of State would remain ultimately accountable for the NHS.

Clegg boasted to a private meeting of his MPs and peers that their demands had been 'very, very handsomely met'. Cameron bolstered this view with his statement: 'I think in politics you have to be big enough to admit when you don't get it right, and that's exactly what I've done.' Clearly, the Conservatives felt they might be taking back the agenda, and it was rumoured that the influential backbench Conservative 1922 Committee had 'cheered Lansley to the rafters' when he announced that the bill was still on track.

Not all Lib Dems were convinced. In June 2011 the *Guardian*'s Wintour and Watt blog revealed a leaked email from Evan Harris in which he told his party colleagues that: 'There is a view that we should keep quiet, say we had a victory and hope no one notices this stuff – but I think that is not realistic. The plans remain bad for the NHS, go beyond the coalition agreement and we must insist on the sovereignty of [our] conference on major issues not in the coalition agreement.' But, as shown by voting figures in subsequent months, this unease did not translate into real opposition.

On 21 June 2011 the pause was ended and the bill went back to the Commons. Simon Burns MP, the Conservative Health Minister, opened the debate at the dispatch box. Responding to an open letter of complaint signed by 85,000 people, Burns called the members of the campaigning group 38 Degrees, 'zombies'.[18] He further commented: 'As Professor Steve Field said in the Future Forum report: "It is time for the pause to end." Professor Field is not alone in the opinion that now is the time to move forward and to enable proper and thorough scrutiny of those parts of the Bill that will change but without delaying the Bill's passage beyond what is absolutely necessary.'

Voices began to call for urgent action on the legislation. The Academy of Medical Royal Colleges, in its official response to the Future Forum report, said: 'We hope the Government will now accept the Future Forum's recommendations in full and move swiftly to make the changes to the Bill and the proposals that are required.' The King's Fund also emphasised the need to avoid unnecessary delay: 'The "pause" has served the NHS, its staff and patients well.'

The other side was regrouping as well. On 9 October 2011 a protest organised by the campaign group UK Uncut took place on Westminster Bridge just outside Parliament. An estimated two thousand health workers and activists attended the protest, causing significant disruption to central London but attracting little if any attention from the media.

COLLABORATORS

The tortuous progress of the bill through Westminster next moved to the House of Lords. There, on 12 October 2011, Lord Owen made a significant attempt to derail the bill. Originally trained as a doctor, and a former Labour Health Minister in the 1970s, Lord Owen was by now a cross-bencher in the Lords, and had already described the bill as 'fatally flawed'. Using a mechanism to refer the legislation to a Select Committee for detailed analysis, Lord Owen argued for further scrutiny of the powers of the NHSCB, the role of Monitor and the duties of the Secretary of State. In the ensuing debate, the 'reforms' came under sustained attack from many of the one hundred peers who queued up to speak.

Among them were fertility doctor and television presenter Lord Winston, who denounced Lansley's bill as 'unnecessary and, I'm afraid to say, irresponsible'. Labour's deputy leader in the Lords, Lord Hunt of Kings Heath, intoned: 'The scale of concern, the scale of mistrust amongst the NHS and amongst the public is greater than I have ever known it before.' But former Conservative Health Secretary Lord Fowler claimed it would be 'unacceptable' for peers to block the legislation. He warned: 'Unless we are careful, we will leave the health service in uncertainty about the future. We will leave them in suspended animation. I don't believe that anyone who is committed to the National Health Service wants to see that.' And the emollient Conservative Lord Howe attempted to calm fears that the extension of market mechanisms which the bill threatened would undermine the founding principles of the NHS: 'The Bill does not do anything that may or could lead to the privatisation of the NHS.' Reform was needed, he said, adding: 'Money will no longer grow on trees in the NHS, we have to think outside of the box.'

Lord Owen's amendment failed to pass, by a margin of 262 to 330, with 193 Tories voting against it, joined by 80 Lib Dem peers. Baroness Williams, who had been a leading Lib Dem opponent of the health bill, did not vote.

Williams, once thought of as a staunch defender of a publicly provided NHS, had turned down an opportunity to take a stand against the bill. Many people felt let down by her failure to vote at this crucial stage. She repeatedly spoke out for the NHS but when it came to voting would fall in line and follow her Lib Dem colleagues in supporting the Conservatives. She had said only a few weeks earlier:

> I am not against a private element in the NHS, which may bring innovatory ideas and good practice, provided it is within the framework of a public service – complementary but not wrecking. But why have they tried to get away from the NHS as a public service, among the most efficient, least expensive and fairest anywhere in the world? Why have they been bewitched by a flawed

> US system, which is unable to provide a universal
> service and is very expensive indeed? The remarkable
> vision of the 1945 Attlee government – of a public
> service free at the point of need for all of the people
> of England – should not be allowed to die.[19]

In a last attempt to derail the bill, Lord Rea, a Labour peer and former practising doctor, tried to deny it a second reading, but his move failed by a margin of 220 to 354. Indeed, even Williams voted against Lord Rea's motion, further disappointing her supporters and opponents of the bill.

The *Guardian*'s social affairs editor, Randeep Ramesh, noted: 'The Lib Dem leadership, which has already signalled amendments will be accepted, have now dipped their hands in the blood of the NHS bill. It might be a stain that is hard to rub off.'[20]

BACKLASH

During this period, one doctor chose a particularly poignant way of highlighting the dangers of Lansley's bill. Dr Clive Peedell, a consultant clinical oncologist in Yorkshire and a member of the BMA Council, was an active opponent of the bill from the outset. Between 10 and 15 January 2012, Peedell and his consultant colleague Dr David Wilson ran the 160 miles from the statue of Aneurin Bevan in Cardiff to Richmond House, London, the headquarters of the DoH, the equivalent of a marathon for each day. At times the going was very tough. A stop in Witney, Oxfordshire, David Cameron's constituency, provided an opportunity for a rally in front of local people in order to highlight the dangers of the proposed Health and Social Care Act – and encouragement. When Peedell and Wilson arrived at Richmond

House on 15 January, a huge crowd greeted their speeches (and painful blisters) with many cheers.

Other organisations had come forward to oppose the bill. These included the NHS Consultants' Association and the NHS Support Federation. Keep Our NHS Public (KONP), a group founded by campaigners to resist the commercialisation of the NHS, also campaigned throughout the entire period, and 38 Degrees organised petitions and sought public support for a legal opinion about the bill, with 3,652 members donating money for this effort at an average donation of £15. It was enough. In the summer of 2011 38 Degrees procured an opinion from solicitors Harrison Grant and specialist barristers Stephen Cragg and Rebecca Haynes.[21] Their reading was that the bill would remove ministerial accountability for the NHS, in effect allowing politicians to wash their hands of any decision making or problems when it came to the health of the nation's citizens. The NHS, the legal experts said, would be opened up to UK and EU competition law, meaning that contracts would have to be offered to the private sector at the same time as they were offered to the NHS – a significant change from the long-standing practice of giving public providers an initial bidding period. The costly and complex procurement procedures appeared to favour large multinational companies, which were more likely to have the resources to submit tenders as compared to smaller NHS or public sector charities. It amounted to a damning indictment of the bill, but it did not seem to attract any attention among Coalition leaders.

A debate had been secured by the Labour front bench in the House of Commons for 13 March 2012 in response to a petition, entitled 'Drop the health bill', which had been launched on the HM Government's e-petition website by NHS campaigner and GP Dr Kailash Chand.[22] When petitions on the HM Government site attract more than 100,000 signatures, Parliament will consider debating them, and this petition, with the backing of 38 Degrees, collected 179,459 signatures.

The subsequent debate was heated. Labour health spokesman Andy Burnham announced: 'I think that Government Members are misjudging the mood of the country, and particularly of health professionals, who have not given a knee-jerk political response to the Bill but have given it careful consideration since it began as a White Paper and then proceeded on its tortuous path through Parliament. They have come to the conclusion that it is better, even now, to abandon it and work back through the existing legal structures of the NHS rather than proceed with the new legal structure and all the upheaval that that entails.'

Lansley responded with an empty reassurance: 'There is nothing in the Bill that creates a free-for-all. There is nothing in it that creates a market of that kind.'

Chris Skidmore, Tory MP, quoted Professor Julian Le Grand of the London School of Economics, a former senior policy adviser to Tony Blair, when he addressed his fellows in the House: 'With respect to the NHS bill, it is important that even those who generally prefer to rely upon their intuitions should avoid muddying the waters by accusing the bill of doing things that it does not, like privatising the NHS; and that all those involved should acknowledge the peer-reviewed evidence demonstrating that its provisions with respect to public competition … are likely to improve patient care.'

When the vote was finally taken, the 'Stop the bill' motion lost by 260 to 314 votes.

Meanwhile, the government persisted in claiming that the problem lay not in the legislation but in the way it had been presented to the medical professions and the public. Lansley was criticised for being a poor communicator. It was the medium, not the message. In the House of Lords Tory Earl Howe, a hereditary peer and former banker as well as a Health Minister, made a revealing comment on 13 March 2012: 'The Government are undoubtedly fighting a battle to convince the medical community of the merits of the Bill, a battle that we have so far not won.' But the urbane peer had for once got it wrong. It was not the salesmanship that the public didn't like, it was the contents of the package, and no amount of marketing skill would alter that.

Further debates occurred in the Lords, culminating on 19 March, when there were calls to make public the Risk Register relating to the bill. This document – a standard way of assessing planned new laws – addresses concerns with their potential impact, of particular importance in the case of the NHS, which by definition deals with matters of life and death. Many campaigners had asked for the Risk Register to be released, but to no avail. A request under the Freedom of Information Act had even been instigated by then Shadow Health Minister John Healey but the request had been vetoed by the government – only the fourth time this had occurred in a decade. This was despite a judge-led information tribunal ordering the DoH to release the document. Andy Burnham said that the veto decision was 'a major step backwards towards secrecy and closed government'. The public just assumed that release of the document would confirm that the warnings from doctors, nurses, midwives and patients were echoed in private by civil servants.

Lord Owen tried again to use the democratic process to bring the Risk Register to light, putting forward a motion asking for the legislation's progress through Parliament to be halted until it was published. A typical intervention came from cross-bencher Baroness Murphy, who had worked as a professor of psychiatry of old age. In the debate, she said: 'The risk register is a complete red herring and we all know that this is an attempt to delay the implementation of the policies in the Bill.' It later transpired that

Baroness Murphy is a former non-executive director for Monitor, the body that was already set to oversee the foundation trusts and that would be the economic regulator of the new open-to-all health care market.

Former BMA president Lord Walton had been an outspoken opponent of the bill, but he said he could not back Lord Owen's push to have the Risk Register released. Among other things, Lord Walton said that the amended bill was much better than it had been when first introduced. 'It is time to give this Bill a third reading', he commented. Given his previous stance, his contribution to the debate could not be easily dismissed.

The Owen motion lost by 213 to 328 votes. The Lib Dems lined up behind their Tory counterparts and none backed Lord Owen. Instead 73 Lib Dem peers voted with the Conservative-led Coalition to block any further delay to the progress of Lansley's bill. The public and most politicians still didn't know what risks were associated with the bill, though the independent Information Commissioner thought they should know. Once again, Baroness Williams failed to vote on this crucial motion.

With the last hurdle passed, the final debate in the Lords began mid-evening. There were many impassioned contributions. Lord Dubs, a Czech-born Jew who had fled the Nazis during the Second World War, stood out with his statement:

> My Lords, I shall speak very briefly as the House wants to move to a vote. I support this amendment and would like to pay a tribute to my noble friend Lady Thornton for the work that she and her team have put into this. Without the backing of a government department, they have performed heroically and very effectively ...
> I want to give only one personal reminiscence. The National Health Service started on 5 July 1948. I was a

child in hospital on that day; I was quite ill in Stockport Royal Infirmary. The consultant and his team came; in those days one either had to stand to attention or lie to attention when the consultant came with the matron and the team of junior doctors. Momentarily, he stopped at the foot of my bed and I said, 'Are we going to celebrate? Are we having a party?' He asked, 'What are you talking about?' I was the only child in the ward, so it was cheeky of me but I said, 'Well, the hospital is ours today – isn't it wonderful?' He walked on without saying anything, but it was a momentous day and I never thought that, 64 years later, I would be here at Westminster and lamenting what has happened to our beloved National Health Service. Let me conclude by quoting Nye Bevan, who said, 'The NHS will last as long as there are folk … with the faith to fight for it.'

The vote came at 8.20p.m. Andrew Lansley and his deputy, Simon Burns, were watching intently from the gallery, wondering if their bill would succeed. The result came a mere fourteen minutes later by a margin of 269 to 174 in support of the Health and Social Care Bill. Baroness Williams voted in favour of the bill. Many would see this vote as the ultimate betrayal of the NHS. For all the fine words that Williams had uttered in the months leading up to this moment, these activists felt that she had failed them when it most mattered.

FINALE

With the battle in the Lords over, the bill was returned to the House of Commons on Tuesday, 20 March 2012, for the final push. Ahead of the debate, Tory and Lib Dem ministers reportedly 'banged' the table at a Cabinet meeting to mark the impending passing of the NHS reforms into law. Labour used this day to say it would repeal the bill if it formed the next government. The bill had received more scrutiny than any bill in living memory and had been amended more than one thousand times, though the vast majority of amendments were trivial.

That evening three debates were heard. During each the major concerns about the bill were reiterated. These concerns included the increased use of the private sector, allowing foundation trusts to undertake more private work, the role of the Secretary of State in the NHS being diminished, the overbearing and powerful influence of Monitor and the NHSCB, and the massive reorganisation of the NHS. At 10p.m. the vote was held. The Conservatives voted as one and the Liberal Democrats followed the Conservatives through the lobby like sheep. The only exception was Greg Mulholland, Lib Dem MP for Leeds North West, who opposed the bill. The final vote was lost by 324 votes to 236.

The Health and Social Care Act would now be sent to Her Majesty Queen Elizabeth II for royal assent, which was given on 27 March 2012. Members of Unison, which represents more than a million public sector workers, held a minute's silence outside Parliament in protest at the legislated changes.

The arrogance of those in power was neatly summed up by one Department of Health civil servant: 'Everybody is a bit bored with talking about the processes and structures.'

Would Aneurin Bevan have been bored talking about the process of the bill and the structures of the NHS? Or would he now be turning in his grave?

4

THE SILENCE OF THE LAMBS

Jacky Davis and David Wrigley

The road to hell is paved with bad excuses.

The Killing

On 27 March 2012 Lansley's Health and Social Care Act finally passed into law. This unwanted and unwieldy piece of legislation had been denounced by every major organisation representing health care workers and had degenerated from a bill to 'empower' doctors with decision making and money to one battling the supposed vested interests of the health care professions. By the time the bill was passed, it had proved unacceptable to the vast majority of doctors and other health workers. So why, on the day of its passage, was Lansley still claiming that he had the backing of doctors? How had his bill survived the critics' mauling and passed on to the statute book? A large part of the responsibility must lie with the behaviour of the medical establishment whose silence, combined with a lack of leadership and timely opposition, undoubtedly allowed the Coalition to get away with this great betrayal of the NHS.

What constitutes the 'medical establishment' and who is capable of wielding the power that should have been used on behalf of the nation's doctors and their patients? The two organisations that would surely be nominated by doctors and those watching medical politics are the British Medical Association (BMA) and the Academy of Medical Royal Colleges (the umbrella organisation for the various medical royal colleges). Between them, these two organisations look after the trade union and professional interests of 250,000 doctors and, as such, have huge potential to influence decisions regarding the NHS. How did they use this power when confronted by Lansley's bill, the biggest challenge to the profession and our patients for decades?

CRITICAL DISENGAGEMENT

The BMA is the foremost of the doctors' trade unions, representing the majority of doctors – a total of 150,000 members. It negotiates on behalf of the profession, claiming to be 'the voice for doctors and medical students throughout the UK'. It also has an important professional role beyond its trade union function, promoting 'the medical and allied sciences and the aims of quality health care'. It is looked to for leadership not only by doctors but also by other health care unions and professional bodies, which realise that the size of the BMA's membership means it has the power to back up its positions, should it choose to do so. So how did the most powerful doctors' trade union square up to the challenge of the Health and Social Care Bill?

The BMA prides itself on being a democratic organisation, with policy decided at its Annual Representative Meeting (ARM).

During the ARM, around four hundred BMA representatives meet to debate issues relevant to doctors. Motions are submitted many weeks in advance. For the June 2010 meeting, Secretary of State for Health Andrew Lansley was given a platform to address this gathering for forty-five minutes. He was heard politely and answered some pre-selected questions. No conference debate on his speech was scheduled, and a request for an emergency debate on the anticipated proposals for GP commissioning was turned down. Under normal circumstances there would be no further opportunity for representatives to debate and produce policy about these changes until the following year's meeting, by which time, many felt certain, any legislation was likely to have been passed.

Less than two weeks later, on 12 July, Lansley launched his White Paper, 'Equity and excellence: Liberating the NHS', which contained proposals with huge implications for the NHS, doctors and patients. The government must have been delighted that the timing of the White Paper meant that it had not been discussed by hundreds of politically active doctors at the June BMA conference.

At the first BMA council meeting after the White Paper's debut, in July 2010, Dr Hamish Meldrum, chair of council, said that it would be folly not to get engaged with the bill, describing it as a 'curate's egg'. He unfortunately missed the irony of the metaphor, as a member soon pointed out in a letter to *BMA News*: 'I venture that BMA Council chairman Hamish Meldrum's assessment that many consider the NHS white paper to be "something of a curate's egg" may be entirely accurate. Those familiar with the origins of the phrase will know that a partly spoiled egg is completely spoiled.' Sadly, this letter was to prove correct.

At that council meeting a small minority spoke out against the White Paper's proposals, arguing that if they were to go ahead, it would lead to the privatisation of the NHS. An emergency motion was passed asking for support for the eight principles of 'Look after our NHS', the anti-privatisation campaign that the BMA was already running. There was also a call for an emergency Special Representatives Meeting so that grass-roots members of the BMA could be allowed the opportunity to debate Lansley's proposals, but this was rejected. Another motion, overwhelmingly passed, called for the BMA to pursue a policy of 'critical engagement' with the government. This policy was pursued with dogged and increasingly misplaced persistence from July 2010 until November 2011, when the BMA leadership was finally forced to move to a position of opposition.

On 30 July 2010 Hamish Meldrum published an open letter to the profession, still using the unfortunate curate's egg analogy. While expressing some concern at more market-based policies (which were in direct contradiction to the BMA's 'Look after the NHS' campaign), he described the proposals as 'an opportunity for doctors to take more control over their working lives and design of services for their patients'.[1] The newsletter *Healthcare Republic* (now GP Online) headlined a piece about the letter: 'Doctors urged not to panic …'.[2] Meldrum was presumably referring to GPs and not to all doctors in the NHS, as remarkably and worryingly there was very little reference in the White Paper itself to the role of hospital doctors. In fact, the White Paper contained very little about hospitals at all.

Soon after, at an 18 August 2010 roundtable discussion of BMA GP leaders exploring the commissioning proposals with key 'stakeholders', the pattern was set, with this group taking charge of the BMA's response to the health bill. The powerful GP Committee, chaired by London GP Dr Laurence Buckman, was to take the lead on the bill, issuing numerous guidance documents and practical suggestions as to how GP consortia (later renamed as clinical commissioning groups ([CCGs][3]) could be set up, and how GPs should get involved in the new structures, even though no legislation had yet been passed. The deputy chair of the GP Committee, Dr Richard Vautrey, enthused that 'GPs will not only bring a perspective that is closer to the patients … but also will have cost effectiveness of service redesign clearly in mind … It also means doing less in hospital and more clinical work in the community'.[4] Both these predictions would later come back to bite when GPs discovered that CCGs were effectively being assigned the role of rationing boards, and that their workload was soaring as care moved into the community without the necessary infrastructure in place. (By June 2012 Vautrey had changed his tune, claiming, 'I do not like the Health and Social Care Act, I think it has the potential to damage the fundamentals of the NHS we all so cherish.'[5] Unfortunately, his conversion came too late.)

But while BMA GP leaders were pressing ahead and encouraging their members to embrace commissioning, many others were less sanguine and alarm bells were being sounded. In September 2010 Unison, which labelled the bill 'a disaster of Titanic proportions', produced a strong critique of the White Paper in the pamphlet 'More than just a brand'.[6] An impressive and sobering read in retrospect, it reveals how quickly some analysts understood the dangers of the proposed 'reforms'. Among other concerns it listed the larger role for the private sector, the opening up of EU competition law, decreased accountability and patient voice, spiralling transaction costs and administrative burden, a postcode lottery and years of expected instability for the NHS. It pointed out that there was no mandate and no evidence base to support the reforms, which, Unison said, were driven by ideology. The report also predicted that care would soon be based on ability to pay, and that the NHS as 'brand name' would be attached to competing *private* services. But of special interest to doctors, 'More than just a brand' drew attention to the likely problems that would arise from the plans to hand NHS budgets and commissioning powers to GPs. Unison, less seduced by the siren call of commissioning than the BMA, warned that commissioning had already proved an expensive failure, having cost hundreds of millions more than it had saved. It also cited an early doctors.net survey,[7] which showed that two-thirds of doctors did not welcome the government's plans and that a similar percentage objected to compulsory participation in consortia,[8] not a good omen for the support from the profession that Andrew Lansley claimed – and needed. Unison also gave a further stark warning, saying that the White Paper threatened national pay bargaining, and with it national terms and conditions for NHS staff, and pointing out that that the proposals explicitly promised a reduction in NHS staff numbers.

Similar warnings were published by organisations such as Keep Our NHS Public (KONP) and London Health Emergency (LHE). Like Unison, LHE predicted fragmentation and privatisation of the NHS, and that CCGs would serve as rationing boards. They also mentioned yet another poll that showed lack of support for Lansley's plan, this one recording that 60 per cent of the entrepreneurial GP members of the National Association of Primary Care (NAPC) – a group more likely to welcome such 'reforms' – were against the commissioning plans. LHE quoted Dr Michael Dixon, a noted cheerleader for Lansley's White Paper, appealing to GPs not to turn their backs on the proposals. The organisation noted that the BMA had not formally spelled out its reservations nor 'identified any issues which might persuade negotiators to pull out if not resolved'. The front page of LHE's 'White Paper special issue' stated in large print: 'If the NHS Alliance, the Royal College of GPs and the BMA, along with the health unions simply took a firm stand against the WP, the ConDems would not be able to carry out their plans.'[9] Unfortunately, few of the organisations addressed were listening, and none appeared to take the advice on board.

The government's 'consultation' on the White Paper was not, as Unison wryly noted, on whether the reforms were the right ones but merely about how they should be implemented. As it was already apparent that many doctors did not welcome the changes, including many of the GPs who seemed most likely to benefit from them, it might have been wise, therefore, for the BMA to gauge the views of the profession before deciding on how to respond. However, the BMA submitted its response to the White Paper without having conducted a survey of its members' opinions. While their submission listed many specific concerns, there was no overall opposition expressed to the proposals, and indeed the BMA asked that 'the pace of change in developing commissioning must allow the vanguard to develop swiftly'.[10] Meanwhile, critics of the 'reforms' within BMA Council were still submitting further motions to get an emergency meeting, which again were rejected or voted down.

In December 2010 the Government published its implementation plan in the form of 'Liberating the NHS: Legislative framework and next steps'. Few if any of the profession's concerns had been taken on board and Meldrum commented that 'nothing much had changed … there was virtually no tangible response to the consultation'.[11] In mid-December the BMA had even issued a press release expressing their disappointment: 'There is little evidence in this response that the government is genuinely prepared to engage with constructive criticism of its plans for the NHS. Most of the major concerns that doctors and many others have raised about the white paper seem, for the most part, to have been disregarded.'[12]

In January 2011 the *British Medical Journal* (*BMJ*) published an open letter from Dr Clive Peedell (the member of the BMA Council who, as already mentioned in chapter 3, would later run the 160 miles from the statue of Aneurin Bevan in Cardiff to Richmond House, London, the headquarters of the Department of Health), which was co-signed by more than one hundred doctors.[13] Addressed to Drs Meldrum and Buckman and the members of the GP Committee, the letter criticised the BMA leadership for continuing the policy of critical engagement when it was already apparent that it was ineffectual. The signatories also took the BMA, and more specifically the BMA General Practitioners Committee, to task for treating proposals in Lansley's White Paper as if they were already policy and for not engaging with the BMA membership. It also pointed out – most importantly – that the BMA had it in its power to successfully oppose the changes: 'From an influence point of view the BMA is critical because it could derail the coalition's white paper reforms, which propose a clinically led system. If the BMA were to say no, then the whole initiative could grind to a halt.' The letter attracted an unprecedented number of rapid responses – more than one hundred – the vast majority of which were supportive. It was also discussed at the prestigious Academy of Medical Royal Colleges; however, it was dismissed there as 'not very well written' and 'alarmist'.

In the face of the letter and a separate grass-roots campaigning initiative, the BMA Council finally agreed to an emergency Special Representatives Meeting, which took place on 15 March 2011.[14] By this time, the Health and Social Care Bill had been published, and it was becoming all too obvious that Andrew Lansley was not prepared to listen. There had been six thousand responses to the White Paper during the 'consultation' period, the responses coming from virtually every representative body across the medical professions, trade unions, patients' organisations and public health experts, and all were overwhelmingly critical. But few, if any, of the profession's concerns were being addressed. Ominously, the seventy-five mentions of GPs in the White Paper contrasted with only a handful in the draft legislation, raising questions about whether GPs would actually have any role in commissioning.

Despite the fact that the BMA had failed to wring a single significant concession from the government, Meldrum told the assembled Special Representatives Meeting that 'critical engagement' was still the right approach. He appealed to the angry delegates packed into the hall not to 'tie the hands of the BMA negotiators', and asked them to reject a motion for all-out opposition to the health bill and also a vote of no confidence in Lansley. Both motions were thus lost at his direction, albeit by a narrow margin.[15] At the same time, and to everyone's confusion, a motion was passed calling for withdrawal of the bill. This resulted in the bizarre situation of the BMA having adopted a policy of calling for the bill to be withdrawn while, at the behest of the leadership, not opposing it.

In the face of mounting concern, the government announced the 'listening' pause on 4 April. In June, the Future Forum published its report and the BMA issued another press release, this time with such rapidity that many assumed the leadership was already privy to the report's findings. Meldrum talked of 'significant revisions' having been made to the bill. The BMA press release quoted him as saying, 'But if the Government does accept the recommendations we have heard today we will be seeing, at the least, a dramatically different Health and Social Care Bill and one that would get us onto a much better track.'[16]

In rapid-fire mode, Dr Michelle Drage, the influential leader of London's GPs, announced that she did not agree. She tweeted: 'Well well well – cop-outs galore raise more questions than answers. This gets more opaque, cumbersome and unaffordable with every utterance.'[17] Likewise, Dr Evan Harris, the influential Liberal Democrat former GP, dismissed the NHS Future Forum report as 'cliché-ridden, trite nonsense' and, according to a report in the *Independent*, 'held out the prospect of further revolts'.[18]

While the BMA was claiming 'significant revisions', Lansley was reassuring his colleagues that the core principles of his reforms remained intact. Both could not be true. And, one by one, most of the BMA's 'significant revisions', in particular reassurances about cherry-picking of services by private health care providers and the role of regulator Monitor in promoting competition, were dropped, falling quietly by the wayside.[19] Lansley was correct when he reportedly promised his backbenchers that no Tory red lines had been crossed.[20]

Despite the BMA's new policy of calling for the bill's withdrawal, Meldrum seemed to think that it was time to 'accept' the proposals and get on with it. On 15 June, speaking at a commissioning conference, he suggested that it was time 'to move on. The time for listening and reflecting [has passed], I think it's now time for doing.'[21] His call was echoed by Professor Steve Field, chair of the Future Forum: 'It is now time for action. The time for politics is over. Clinical leadership is the way forward.'[22]

By now, the bill's critics inside the BMA were starting to ask about 'Plan B', the fall-back position that should be taken if and when the called-for 'significant amendments' did not materialise. Questions were asked about lines in the sand. What would happen if the Government remained intransigent and pushed the bill through, warts and all? The concerns fell on deaf ears and the BMA leadership's only policy remained that of 'critical engagement', with all this massive organisation's negotiating eggs still stubbornly tucked inside one basket.

The calendar had moved forward one year, and it was time for the BMA's Annual Representative Meeting once again, which in theory would give the grass-roots membership the opportunity to debate the bill – and suggest what to do about it. The meeting was scheduled to take place in Cardiff from Monday, 27 June, to Thursday, 30 June 2011. However, the published agenda was a disappointment. Many of the submitted motions criticising the bill were not listed for debate, and, worse still, fifteen motions calling for withdrawal or opposition to the bill were listed in the 'grey area' – that is, they were also not up for debate. The agenda committee had not scheduled a single motion that would allow this purportedly representative body to debate calling for withdrawal or opposition to the bill. In addition, the whole topic was moved from the Monday, the traditional day for NHS-related debates, to the last day of the conference, by which time most of the media would have likely packed their bags and the delegates would already be drifting home.

BMA representatives then discovered that Meldrum was due to appear before the parliamentary public bill committee on the afternoon of Tuesday, 28 June, before they had had a chance to discuss the bill. Desperate behind-the-scenes manoeuvres resulted in an emergency motion calling for the bill to be withdrawn, a motion that came before the ARM on Tuesday morning. Once again, Meldrum appealed to the representatives to reject the motion for withdrawal, even though this was already established as BMA policy. Once again they ignored him and the motion was passed with a significant majority.

Later in the day Meldrum appeared before the parliamentary committee by video link and was asked why his members kept voting for withdrawal of the bill, against his recommendation. His answer implied to the MPs that the BMA conference delegates did not understand the complex bill, an uncomplimentary assertion that was challenged by one of the MPs, who said he thought that BMA members were of 'average or above-average intelligence'.[23] Meldrum claimed afterwards that there had been errors in the transcription, but an analysis of the records showed no significant mistakes.[24] Whatever his exact words, Meldrum had not given a fair picture of the debate at the BMA conference, during which no one had claimed to be confused by the bill. Some of the representatives, steeped in the details of the byzantine bill, resented the perceived slur. Tempers ran high and there were public protests, including an accusation by Professor Wendy Savage that Meldrum had not told the truth to the parliamentary committee. Pandemonium broke out and the accusation was graciously withdrawn under pressure after it was pointed out that misleading a parliamentary committee was a criminal offence. But the fact remained – Meldrum had failed to use his appearance as an opportunity to put the case against the bill that had been so clearly rehearsed by his members earlier in the day and, what's more, had implied that they simply did not get it. At this stage, the gap between the position of the BMA leadership and its members was looking uncomfortably wide.

Shortly afterwards BMA Council passed a motion for a public campaign for withdrawal of the bill. The proposed campaign was reported in the *BMJ*,[25] alongside a quote from Meldrum stating that, 'it really would be better if the bill were withdrawn', a statement oddly reminiscent of those old notices in Harrods saying 'we would prefer it if you didn't smoke'. But, despite these fighting words, nothing materialised that looked remotely like a campaign, and BMA members began to ask why. Meldrum told an irate meeting in London that he had been advised that there should be no campaign as these had not been effective in the past. After angry internal exchanges he told a BMA council member that he personally had taken a decision not to sanction 'a significant public campaign'. The leadership had apparently decided for whatever reason that there was to be no public campaign despite its own council calling for one.

On 6 September, the day of the third reading of the bill, Meldrum co-signed, with representatives of the Royal College of GPs and the Royal College of Nursing, a letter to *The Times* calling for further 'significant amendments' but with no mention of a call for withdrawal of the bill. Things started to grow more serious for the leadership when a regional meeting of BMA London members passed a motion of censure against Meldrum for not organising a campaign. Their move reflected the feelings of many that the BMA was rapidly losing touch with its grass roots. *Pulse* magazine quoted 'a BMA source' as saying, 'Hamish is furious about being censured but it reflects the failure of the BMA's "critical engagement" policy on the health bill. In any other walk of life where you pushed a policy for a year and it turned out to be a complete failure you would at least admit it was wrong and do something stronger, particularly when your members are mandating you to do so … They will rally round Hamish at Council level but the problem is the ordinary member doesn't have a voice that Hamish can hear. The London branch might have become that.'[26]

The BMA Council did indeed rally round, with a vote of support for Meldrum. Council members were reminded that they must accept principles of collective responsibility, and were warned of possible expulsion if they didn't. The atmosphere was decidedly unpleasant.

In November a new Department of Health document about commissioning made it clear that most key commissioning functions would be performed by 'commissioning support units', contracted by CCGs and to be outsourced to the private sector by 2015.[27] This was a significant change in approach, and a devastating shift for those GPs who still believed they were going to be given the power to shape services. It proved the last straw for many. The BMA Council finally passed a motion, proposed by the authors of this chapter, calling for opposition to the entire bill, a position resisted for so long by the BMA leadership. The motion also called for 'a significant public campaign', but this was yet again ignored in the coming months – unless you count an online Christmas card and an online day of action which saw the NHS trending in the UK's Top 15 issues on Twitter as a campaign to save the NHS.

The BMA and its membership were by now looking at a complete betrayal by Lansley. Laurence Buckman, head of the GP Committee, sent out a letter expressing his concern and disappointment: 'We firmly believe that the balance is tipping against clinicians having any real influence over commissioning and that the direction of travel now risks more than we thought we stood to gain from clinically led commissioning.'[28]

Yet in the face of this treachery Buckman's committee ruled out one source of effective action: they would not ask GPs to withdraw from commissioning.[29] No one thought to consult the forty thousand GPs in England as to whether they agreed with the decision. BMA leaders sought an urgent meeting with Lansley, but in the absence of any credible threat from their side there was no shift in the government's position. The situation remained unchanged. The bill had not yet passed into law, but it was beginning to look like game, set and match to Lansley.

In December 2011 the BMA at long last published a briefing paper, 'Why the BMA is opposing the whole bill',[30] with the objective that the bill should be 'abandoned'. The paper studiously avoided mentioning the threat of privatisation, though this was one of the biggest concerns surrounding the legislation, and instead focused on 'chaos' on the ground, particularly objections to the 'speed and pace' of reforms and the complexity of the bill. With this last feeble gasp, the BMA leadership turned with relief to the vexed question of the attack on doctors' pensions, a fight they were unlikely to win as a result of failing to stand up to Lansley over the 'reforms'. 'New leadership is needed at the BMA', tweeted Richard Smith, one-time editor of *BMJ*, over the pensions debacle.[31] By this stage, many agreed.

THE COMPLICIT ENABLERS

The second pillar of the medical establishment is the Academy of Medical Royal Colleges, an umbrella organisation for the various medical royal colleges. These venerable bodies, some dating back centuries, represent the different medical specialities and their remit is medical training and standards of clinical care. But their influence is much wider and deeper.

For example, the Royal College of Surgeons states on its website that the organisation 'provide[s] strategic leadership by engaging at the highest level with Government, the Department of Health, national and local commissioners, Trusts, regulatory and professional bodies to influence national healthcare policy. As a professional body the College is uniquely placed to demonstrate best surgical practice and to lobby for improved care for patients.'[32] Since Lansley's bill threatened to affect adversely both training and clinical standards, it was to be hoped and expected that the medical royal colleges would have something to say about it, particularly once it became apparent that Lansley intended to ignore the concerns of the profession.

The colleges did indeed produce reams of documents in response to the government's White Paper 'consultation', and again during the 'listening' pause. Many concerns were listed in these documents, but having produced piles of papers the leaders of these venerable institutions seemed to think their job was done. Rather like the BMA, they seemed to believe they could change the government's mind through reason and clinical evidence, backed up with a good dose of 'strenuous lobbying'. After all, Lansley had promised that clinicians would be at the heart of his reforms. This betrayed a fatal political ingenuousness and a misunderstanding of Lansley's rationale for the massive and detailed bill. The colleges appeared to have no plans for what they might do if and when the government turned a deaf ear to them, and almost all failed to consult directly with their own membership.

The one college that did consult its members from the very beginning was the Royal College of General Practitioners (RCGP). In the summer of 2010 their chair was Professor Steve Field, a well-known enthusiast for Lansley's reforms who described them as a 'once-in-a-lifetime chance'[33] for GPs when they were unveiled to the public. His members didn't necessarily agree, and an early RCGP consultation on the White Paper received four hundred responses – an unprecedented outpouring. The overwhelming view in the responses was that 'the bill stank' and that Field's support for it 'did not represent the views of the majority of the profession'. One insider's view was that Field was 'too closely aligned with Andrew Lansley'.

Steve Field came to the end of his term in office at the RCGP in November 2010 and was replaced by Dr Clare Gerada, who was decidedly less enthusiastic about Lansley's bill. An early interview with the *Guardian* that month described her as a 'passionate' critic of the reforms.[34] She began saying in public what others were only prepared to say behind closed doors.

The government could not afford to have the powerful leader of England's forty thousand GPs criticising the bill and immediately set about undermining Gerada. Her public statements, backed by her council, were repeatedly dismissed by ministers despite the fact that the RCGP conducted three surveys and numerous consultations on the bill, far more than any other college. Junior Health Minister for the Tories, Anna Soubry, appearing on BBC Two's *Daily Politics* programme, accused Gerada of only working 'part time'[35] – a stunning show of gendered politics – and Simon Burns, Conservative MP for Chelmsford, infamously remarked 'Oh God'[36] when Gerada's name was mentioned in a parliamentary debate. Gerada was repeatedly patronised not only by ministers but by the predominantly male medical establishment too, with one official of a noticeably reticent college declaring that her position of public opposition was about personal aggrandisement,[37] an accusation that certainly could not be made against other college leaders who mostly had their heads well below the parapet.

Apart from the RCGP, only the Royal College of Psychiatrists surveyed their members to find their views on Lansley's bill. The results consistently showed that over 80 per cent of respondents believed that the bill would have a detrimental effect on the NHS and wanted it withdrawn.

As the government became ever more intransigent and the passage of the bill loomed nearer, college members, who pay significant subscriptions for their membership, began to voice their anxieties. What would happen if the bill went through without the 'significant amendments' that those in charge were still seeking? Why weren't their professional leaders doing more to stop the advance of the legislation?

The last straw for many was reached on 24 January 2012, when the twenty medical royal colleges met with the BMA and the Royal College of Nursing (RCN), both of which were already in declared opposition to the bill. At this point, most of the colleges were still sitting on the fence. By this time they could have been under no illusion about the views of the great majority of doctors. A recent poll of RCGP members had found that 98 per cent would back a call for the health bill to be withdrawn if this was made in tandem with other royal colleges.[38] The chairman of the BMA's GP trainee subcommittee had launched an e-petition, 'Call for Mr Lansley to resign', in a bid to force Parliament to debate whether the Health Secretary should step down over his NHS reform plans.[39] There was no longer any excuse not to act.

Those present knew that the decision before them could not be more important: nothing less than the fate of the NHS was in their hands. Those who knew about the meeting waited anxiously to hear what would emerge. Would the royal colleges withdraw their tacit support for the bill and hasten its demise? For surely the bill – already badly damaged – could not survive a full frontal attack from the united medical establishment.

With the exception of the surgeons, those present agreed to support a draft statement. It was not forceful enough for some and too political for others, but given the spectrum of opinion present in the meeting, it was a significant achievement. At its heart was the all-important declaration: 'The Academy and medical royal colleges are not able to support the bill as it currently stands.'[40]

Before the participants could meet again to ratify the statement, a draft was leaked and the government launched a counter-attack. Ministers phoned college officials, with a flurry of hints coming from several directions that their institutions would be 'out in the cold' for years, that no one would answer their phone calls and that they might lose their cherished charitable status if opposition became official. It was clear that the government was afraid of the combined power of the colleges. It was ready to use both sticks and carrots to get them back in line.

One by one the colleges withdrew their support and the statement that was finally issued proved to be a bathetic anticlimax: 'A number of Medical Royal Colleges, the BMA, the RCN and organisations representing other clinical professionals, met today (26/1/12) to discuss their approaches to the Health and Social Care Bill. There was a useful exchange of information and an agreement to continue the dialogue.'[41]

The elephant had given birth to a mouse.

Lansley and the government must have heaved a huge sigh of relief while the members of the colleges, whose subscriptions keep them in business, wondered what on earth had happened to democracy. There seemed to be no way to express their outrage at this collapse in moral courage, or to light a fire under their august leaders, until someone remembered that the constitutions of all the colleges included a mechanism for calling Extraordinary General Meetings (EGMs).

Anti-bill activists, led by one of this chapter's authors, Dr David Wrigley, rapidly set up a website named Call on Your College, and advertised it widely via social media. The purpose was to collect enough proposers to call for college EGMs. These were quickly achieved for most of the colleges, which required relatively small numbers of signatures to force an EGM. The exception was the Royal College of Paediatrics and Child Health, whose articles and bylaws required six hundred signatures to trigger such a meeting. The requisite signatures were collated, and the colleges informed. The responses to this challenge ranged from the polite to the arrogant, with one of this chapter's authors being told down the phone, 'Well, I've never heard of you!' to which the reply was, 'Well, I've never heard of you either, but you are still obliged to organise an EGM.' One could sense the gold chains of office clanking in indignation, and the vintage port being broken out early, as the EGM outrage was discussed.

Most colleges showed good grace and organised emergency meetings as required by their constitutions. Some dragged their feet for so long that their meetings took place after the bill had been passed. The meetings were well attended given that they were largely held during the day, at short notice and that doctors need six weeks' notice of leave from their practice. With one exception – the Royal College of Surgeons, whose president, Professor Norman Williams, had recently declared, 'The College largely supports the aims of the reforms to modernise the healthcare system'[42] – there were overwhelming votes in support of calling for the bill to be withdrawn. But even this wasn't enough in some cases, with officials reluctantly agreeing to take the motions back to their governing councils for 'consideration'. The great and the good who represent doctors did not appreciate being called to account by them.

Some doctors simply bypassed their colleges – more than four hundred public health doctors wrote an open letter to the Lords, published in the *Telegraph*, rejecting the bill.[43] They cited irreparable harm to the NHS, to individual patients and to society as a whole. Lansley's response was to maintain that the doctors, including more than one hundred leading academics, had signed the letter without reading it, and a DoH spokesman asserted that it was not supported by 'a shred of evidence'[44] – rich coming from a department whose reforms had no evidence base whatsoever.

THE END GAME

The final weeks before the passage of the bill saw more frantic attempts from a handful of politicians and doctors, including Clare Gerada, to organise opposition. In December, Andy Burnham, Shadow Secretary of State for Health, who had already tried to harness various efforts, called a meeting of the colleges and the unions. He attempted to persuade those present that if they all united, the bill could fall. One of those present reported: 'The medical establishment was there and in power but the medics are not going to come out – there is too much self-interest.'

This was followed by yet another leak, and the rapid appearance of an article in the *Guardian* about Labour's 'plan B' opposition to the health bill, hinting that the colleges might not wish to be aligned with what could be perceived as a political initiative.[45] Burnham wrote saying that he was not responsible for the leak, but the suggestion of a link to a political initiative must have frightened the horses and no consensus emerged. Burnham called another meeting in January, still trying to get a united medical front, but two colleges – the RCS and the Royal College of Obstetricians and Gynaecologists (RCOG) – still would not oppose the bill, and once again the initiative failed.

In February 2012, with only a few weeks remaining before the bill was passed, a final 'last stand' was attempted by the RCGP. Yet again, news about the proposed meeting was leaked and the government immediately convened its own Downing Street 'summit', inviting only those 'constructively engaged in implementing the modernisation'.[46] Invitations were sent out on Friday for a meeting on the following Monday, which smacked of indecent haste, perhaps even naked fear. Unfortunately, instead of showing some solidarity, most of those invited turned up for what was reportedly a PR exercise designed to isolate the awkward squad in public, and the meeting itself seemed to serve little purpose except to exclude those in opposition to the bill, including the BMA, the RCN and the RCGP. The *Telegraph* subsequently published a letter from thirty-five members of the Royal College of Physicians saying that their president should have declined the invitation, with one member accusing Sir Richard Thompson of providing 'cover for the Government over its controversial reforms'.[47]

The 'summit' was mostly notable for what went on outside Downing Street, where June Hautot, an outspoken pensioner, door-stepped Lansley and accused him of wanting to privatise the NHS – and of lying about it. The encounter was widely covered by the media, including the BBC. People were delighted that at last someone was speaking the truth to power in the vicinity of Downing Street, recognising perhaps that it would be unwise to rely too much on those lined up inside.

There was some last-minute action, as one by one the various medical organisations publicised their opposition. At this stage the RCN, the RCGP, the Royal College of Midwives (RCM) and the BMA had come out in opposition, as well as those colleges whose hands had been forced by members to do so through the mechanism of the emergency meetings. But piecemeal opposition did not have the same effect as a united front would have done, and already people were focusing their attention elsewhere. The BMA had long ago launched a fight back over pensions (proving they could conduct a public campaign and survey members when it suited them).

When the bill passed, it was burdened with more than one thousand amendments, none of them 'significant'. Lansley boasted that the amendments did not fundamentally change the legislation's core principles. He had, against the odds, managed to get away with it.

THE PRICE OF SILENCE

While the size and contents of Lansley's bill were a surprise to most, it is less clear how much the leaders of the professions knew in advance. None of the proposals appeared in any election manifesto, but they had been trailed in papers and speeches. As one health department official put it: 'There is no excuse for not knowing what the Conservatives were planning to do on health. It must have been one of the most closely pre-advertised plans in history.'[48]

Certainly some in the health policy community were in no doubt. Professor Allyson Pollock, when asked before the 2010 BMA annual conference what three things should be on the agenda, had replied: 'GP commissioning, GP commissioning, GP commissioning.' According to Nicholas Timmins, Laurence Buckman spent 'many hours' with Lansley before the election, and later confirmed that he'd had pre-election talks during which practice-based commissioning had been discussed. When asked what the BMA GP Committee would think about the fact that commissioning was to be compulsory, something that most GPs resented, Lansley is reported to have said, 'I've got them on board.'[49] A member of his team confirmed: 'We genuinely thought they were signed up to the main ideas.'

Indeed, the BMA's own newsletter, *BMA News*, gave a preview of Lansley's White Paper on 3 July 2010, ten days before it was published, when it revealed that GP commissioning would be done against 'a backdrop of huge structural upheaval as primary care organisations and strategic health authorities merge or cease to exist'. Since this aspect of the White Paper was to come as a surprise to most, it seems that the BMA, at least those in the leadership, had some prior knowledge of what was in store. They definitely responded to it quickly. On 18 July, Buckman wrote to all GPs warning of concerns but saying that the GP Committee had already entered discussion with ministers and would help doctors 'rise to the challenge'. The letter was sent out before the BMA Council had even had a chance to discuss its position on the White Paper.

It is perhaps understandable that the BMA opted for 'critical engagement' as a first response, but after the bill was published and it became apparent that the government was ignoring the concerns of the profession, this position became increasingly indefensible. Lansley had a well-deserved reputation for not listening to critics. It seemed highly unlikely that 'intensive lobbying' would result in the 'significant amendments' sought by both the BMA and the colleges. Lansley's bill was lengthier than the original legislation setting up the NHS. It was all of a piece, woven of whole cloth, and it was obvious to most that he was not going to change core features such as the increasing role of competition and the private sector.

The BMA had a long-standing policy of rejecting the privatisation of the NHS, and the eight principles of its 'Look after our NHS' campaign called for co-operation over competition and decreased involvement of the commercial sector. The bill threatened to emphasise competition and accelerate the privatisation of the NHS, but this was apparently deemed of less importance than the holy grail of GP commissioning. Lansley knew what he was doing when he baited the bear trap of his reforms with the tasty morsel of commissioning. Throughout the long and contested passage of the bill, the BMA leadership persisted in the mistaken belief that they could cherry-pick the parts of the reform package that they wanted and reject 'the more damaging aspects'. Even when it became increasingly obvious that the rotten parts of the curate's egg meant that all of it was spoilt, they continued to claim they could still rescue commissioning in a form that suited them.

Most GPs were, of course, afraid of what would happen if they didn't take up the challenge, believing that their more entrepreneurial colleagues would fill the gap. Many letters and papers emerged from BMA headquarters telling the grassroots GPs how to get involved. With greater or lesser enthusiasm they began to organise themselves into consortia. Unfortunately, but predictably, Lansley seized on this as proof that GPs welcomed the Health and Social Care Bill – a claim rejected by the BMA, but the damage was done. GPs, in the absence of any other message from their leaders, had little choice but to go along with the reorganisation even before the bill was passed.

THE CHEERLEADERS

One of the problems for those fighting against the Health and Social Care Bill was the fact that there were cheerleaders for the legislation within the profession, and some undoubtedly did feel, at least in the early days, that the proposed reforms would benefit doctors and patients. Unfortunately, the engagement of an enthusiastic minority allowed the government to claim that doctors were behind the bill right up until the day that the legislation was passed. The fact that by then the number of doctors backing it had dwindled to vanishing point was never exposed by the media.

Some organisations were (and are) explicitly committed to GP commissioning and had the ear of the politicians from the outset. The National Association of Primary Care (NAPC), for instance, contains a mixture of professional and commercial interests, and its partners include Harmoni and UnitedHealth Group UK. NAPC's plans for commissioning met with Tory approval while the party was still in opposition,[50] allowing them to punch well above their weight when Cameron came to power. Its chair, Dr Charles Alessi, a GP in south London, appeared on TV backing the health bill's reforms and wrote effusive articles in outlets such as the *Sun*.[51] When the *Guardian* reported that his practice was found to have 'let go' patients requiring high levels of care, an official investigating the case was quoted: 'I could draw no conclusion other than that you subsequently selected 48 vulnerable people for removal from your list of patients because of their demands on your practice's services and this by virtue of their age, medical condition or level of disability.'[52]

Another organisation that had influence beyond its size was the NHS Alliance, which was also in favour of GP commissioning. Their leader, Dr Michael Dixon, is a 'prime mover in developing GP commissioning' and proponent of complementary medicine (he was for a while the medical director of The Prince's Foundation for Integrated Health, which closed in 2010 after its finance director was arrested for allegedly stealing £253,000 from the organisation[53]). A list of his recent roles is impressive and indicative of how much influence can be gained by those who are able and willing to promote a government's policy.[54] Dixon welcomed the Health and Social Care Bill, saying: 'My short response to it was "wonderful" … it was very emancipating – all that we could have asked for.'

Dr Johnny Marshall, a previous chair of the NAPC, soon emerged as one of the country's strongest voices in favour of the government's NHS reforms.[55] He has since moved onwards and upwards to become an advisory member of the NHS Commissioning Board Authority Future Design Group and an associate director at the NHS Confederation, another pro-privatisation organisation.

Another previous chair of the NAPC who was promoted to greater things is Dr James Kingsland OBE, a 'figure head for commissioning enthusiasts' who had 'a central role in supporting the reform agenda for the NHS'.[56] He was complimented by *Pulse* magazine for the political skill he showed in being 'appointed by the [DoH] to the influential role of special adviser on commissioning, providing him with a direct line to Mr Lansley'. Once again, his list of appointments, both under the Coalition Government and the previous government, is indicative of how influential an individual can be if peddling the right agenda.

Another group that was over-represented during this period was Doctors for Reform, a group of doctors 'supported' by the 'independent think thank' Reform. The officers of Doctors for Reform profess commitment to the values of the NHS while periodically calling for its replacement by a social insurance system with patient charges and more private provision. Despite their small membership – less than a thousand – they were repeatedly interviewed by the media without any reference to their privatisation agenda (as will be detailed in chapter 6).

These organisations and individuals, although being few in number, had a disproportionate influence on both policy and implementation. They allowed the BMA to claim that GPs had to get involved in commissioning, even though the majority didn't want to, because 'if we don't they will'. They were 'the zombie masters', recycling daft ideas that suited no one but the government and themselves.

RESISTANCE IS FUTILE

One obvious solution to the growing concerns was for the BMA simply to oppose the health bill and campaign for its withdrawal, but repeated calls from within the BMA Council to oppose the bill were voted against by the majority of council members and rejected by the leadership right up until November 2011. Many reasons were put forward ranging from 'it's not our job to oppose an elected government' to the more pragmatic 'we can't possibly win the fight'. But the grass roots were overwhelmingly opposed to Lansley's reforms throughout. There was sound evidence from surveys conducted by others that the great majority of doctors did not approve of the bill, or want anything to do with it, but the BMA steadfastly refused to consult its membership. One early survey focused mainly on how people were coping with the proposed changes and what effects the changes would have, but thereafter there was no attempt to harness the voice of tens of thousands of doctors. Some members of council pressed repeatedly for a survey of members, but their requests were turned down. Laurence Buckman told a conference that there was no need for surveys as it was clear the majority of members were overwhelmingly hostile to the bill. The attitude of the leadership was, 'we know what they think.'[57] It would certainly have been a powerful weapon if the

BMA leadership had turned that into public knowledge, but for whatever reason they chose not to. The policy of 'critical engagement' crucially did not extend to their membership.

The BMA was also careful in its criticisms of the bill. It is noteworthy that while the government was very vulnerable to accusations of privatising the service, the BMA studiously avoided using the 'p' word, and indeed their political unit produced a paper proving that what was proposed did not constitute privatisation. Dr Clive Peedell argued in a letter published by the *BMJ* that the proposals fit all the criteria of privatisation, including those of the World Health Organisation,[58] but the BMA never publicly criticised Lansley's repeated statements that the bill was not about privatising the NHS. By failing to use the word, the BMA allowed the government to continue to reject the one criticism that could have caused immense damage with the public.

The other lie that neither the BMA nor the royal colleges challenged publicly was the government's claim about the failings of the NHS. As related elsewhere, when Lansley took over in 2010 the NHS was doing well. Patient and public satisfaction were high and outcomes were improving rapidly after the Labour Government had increased funding.[59] The awkward fact was that the NHS didn't need another 'redisorganisation', and indeed almost everything Lansley claimed he wanted to do could have been achieved without legislation. David Cameron had, on a number of occasions, publicly promised 'no more top-down reorganisations'. The Conservatives needed reasons for betraying their promises and subjecting the NHS to a radical restructure, and so they appear to have made them up. Statistics were cherry-picked and massaged to support claims that the NHS was doing badly – and the media dutifully reported them. As a result, public satisfaction with the service fell sharply – by 12 per cent.[60] The claims should have been analysed and rejected, but it was left to Twitter,[61] and Professor John Appleby, chief economist at

The King's Fund,[62] to expose the lies and half truths. The medical establishment let these assertions go largely unchallenged.

The medical royal colleges are not of course trade unions, but for that very reason their voice is powerful. They cannot be accused of the usual shortcomings of unions: self-interest and protectionism. But they are innately conservative and had not been used to intervening in what they see as 'political' debates. Indeed many leaders expressed fear that the colleges might lose their charitable status if they did so. With the exception of the Royal College of General Practitioners and the Royal College of Psychiatrists, they also neglected to consult their members. It wasn't until their hands were forced that they held emergency meetings to hear what their members wanted them to do. As a result, all but one – the Royal College of Surgeons – had to adopt a position of opposition to the health bill.

Why were the colleges so slow to act and why did their courage fail time and again? Lord David Owen, a fellow of the Royal College of Physicians and one-time Minister of Health, offered this explanation: 'Some of the royal colleges like the RCGP were brave and confident in their criticisms as professional bodies. Others were vacillating and weak. I have no doubt that if the royal colleges had consulted their members early in the process the resultant unease and later backlash would have meant that the "pause" would have become permanent. It was hard to avoid feeling that if not complicit many were afraid of upsetting the Department of Health and afraid of having their financial grants blocked or reduced by running the risk of looking overly political.'[63]

Professor John Ashton, president of the Faculty of Public Health, had harsher words:

> As chair of the Public Health Association when the
> bill was introduced I was prepared to give Clegg the

benefit of the doubt and was one of a small group of senior people including Royal College Presidents who had several meetings with him in the first half of 2011.

However after the 'pause' it became clear to me that the government was acting in bad faith and that the NHS was about to be torn apart by private competition. At that point I could only conclude that some of the senior professionals who continued to collaborate with the bill had been corrupted by the pursuit of honours.[64]

According to Ashton, the Faculty of Public Health was en route to becoming a royal college during this period. However, after members called for opposition to the bill at an emergency general meeting, the application ran into the sand. The faculty's charitable status was investigated, it is rumoured at the instigation of Andrew Lansley.

As for the other unions and professional bodies, it is clear from talking to those present at meetings that everyone, including the TUC, was looking for leadership to the BMA and the Academy of Medical Royal Colleges, but that it was not forthcoming. According to one person who attended several meetings, but who wished to remain anonymous: 'The BMA sat on its hands for far too long over the bill and was either very naive or was trying to get private deals. It came out against the bill far too late and has since been very silent. The BMA had a real opportunity to provide leadership and to mobilise the medical profession against the bill. It never did. Despite our belief in the equality of all those who work in the NHS, it is only when doctors revolt that politicians really listen. At meetings the BMA, alongside the RCN, were arguing for the lowest level of activity.'[65]

It is also clear from Nick Timmins's book *Never Again?* that for a long period the bill was vulnerable to concerted opposition from the professionals who had to implement it. Survey after survey conducted by entities ranging from the BBC to the Nuffield Foundation showed that doctors distrusted and rejected Lansley's reforms. The bill was denounced publicly by the *BMJ* as 'Dr Lansley's Monster',[66] as well as by *The Lancet* ('It's time to kill this Bill'[67]), and doctors and academics wrote hundreds of critical letters and articles. Politicians spoke of 'if' rather than 'when' the bill was passed and at one stage things got so bad there was even talk of whether to 'kill the bill'.[68] A bill that was meant to put clinicians in the driving seat could not survive the united opposition of the medical establishment.

At this crucial moment in the history of the NHS, the doctors' representative bodies proved unable to represent their own members, never mind the interests of their patients. This betrayal of their calling will have damaging consequences for many years to come.

Why was the profession so badly let down by the leadership? Why did those who could and should have acted in concert fail to present a united front? Why was there an over-reliance on the probity of politicians? Why did they continue to depend on 'strenuous lobbying' long after the policy had passed its sell-by date, arguing that it was better to 'stay in the tent'? Why did BMA leaders continue to insist that getting the bill scrapped would be 'an unachievable feat' while failing to mobilise the very professionals who might have achieved that end? Why did they simply refuse to represent their members? Why did our leaders fail the most important challenge the profession has faced in recent memory?

Many theories have been advanced, none of them flattering, and ultimately only the people involved will be able to tell us why they behaved as they did. Thus far there have been no post-mortems and no one involved has expressed any remorse or contrition, or indeed any suggestion that they failed in their duties to represent their members. Not a single leader of the profession has been held to account in any way. Meanwhile, we might like to consider that in medicine, as on the larger stage, 'we get the politicians we deserve'. Through benign neglect, being happy for others to take on these onerous positions on our behalf, doctors ended up with leaders who proved to be complicit enablers, who plainly weren't up to the challenge. The medical profession must learn this lesson for the future.

Finally, it is worth asking what was gained by 'critical engagement' and staying in the tent. It is already apparent that the reward for those who 'engaged' rather than 'opposed' has been 'a really good look at the underside of LaLa's [Lansley's] bulldozer', as Roy Lilley put it on his blog.[69] Less than a year after the bill passed into law, the holy grail of commissioning had already turned to base metal. In the spring of 2013 legislation was put forward to complete the transformation of the NHS into a fully fledged market. Contrary to all the promises made to the profession and the Coalition partners along this long and painful journey, CCGs will be obliged to tender out almost all services or risk expensive legal challenges from the private sector. Clare Gerada recently estimated that only twenty-five GPs in the country are still interested in commissioning.[70]

A few GPs are taking full advantage of the new arrangements, accepting financial incentives to cut back on referrals and prescribing or offering to do privately what was previously available on the NHS.[71] Over a third of GPs on CCGs have conflicts of interests arising from connections with private health care companies[72] and some are already awarding themselves contracts.[73] Dr Mark Porter, leader of the BMA, warned that NHS reforms 'are putting patients' trust in GPs at risk'.[74]

Elsewhere, doctors' morale has 'tumbled',[75] as they 'struggl[e] under the weight of a wholesale NHS reorganisation';[76] CCGs are looking like primary care trusts (PCTs) only with lower management budgets;[77] and even supporters of the reforms are now complaining bitterly that CCGs are 'swamped by red tape'.[78] Or as one GP, Dr Bob Gill, succinctly put it – 'we've got less control, more complexity and all the blame'.

The betrayal of the NHS and the medical profession by the profession is complete.

5

A FAILURE OF POLITICS

Charles West

*The Liberal Democrats exist to build and safeguard
a fair, free and open society, in which we seek to
balance the fundamental values of liberty, equality and
community, and in which no-one shall be enslaved by
poverty, ignorance or conformity … We aim to disperse
power, to foster diversity and to nurture creativity.
We believe that the role of the state is to enable all
citizens to attain these ideals, to contribute fully to their
communities and to take part in the decisions which
affect their lives.*

Preamble, Liberal Democrat Federal Constitution

When the sixty pages of Andrew Lansley's White Paper, and the five supporting documents that followed it, appeared in the summer of 2010, many of the media's headlines proclaimed that £80 billion of the NHS budget would be given over to GPs to spend on behalf of their patients. As a GP with management experience, and a Liberal Democrat, whose party had helped to form the Coalition, you might have expected me to welcome such a proposal. I did not.

It was less than sixty days since the publication of the Coalition agreement, in which David Cameron and Nick Clegg had together promised: 'We will stop the top-down reorganisations of the NHS that have got in the way of patient care.' The Coalition had promised that members of the various primary care trusts (PCTs) would be directly elected. But now, in the White Paper, Lansley was announcing that he was going to abolish not only PCTs but the strategic health authorities (SHAs) too. He claimed to be giving power to patients, GPs and local authorities all at the same time. In my view, these were not small changes, or patient-centred ones. Sir David Nicholson, the chief executive of the NHS, would later call this change programme 'so large that you can see it from outer space'.

Instead of welcoming the White Paper proposals, I felt sure they were set to repeat the mistakes of previous governments. Until the mid-1980s the NHS had been run by a series of committees, most of which were comprised of professional clinicians: a consultant, a senior nurse, a GP, a public health doctor and an administrator. The set-up nearly matched the archetypal 'matron and medical superintendent' that makes modern politicians go all misty-eyed. Had Lansley and his fellow Tory health 'reformers' really wanted to put clinicians in the driving seat, they could have looked to that previous model as a guide.

Even then, long before the current financial crisis, political leaders had worried about the chances that health care spending would spiral out of control. They cited the rising numbers of elderly patients, the increasing complexity of medical technology and the rising expectation of care – the same three fears that reformers cite today. This, despite the findings of the 1979 Royal Commission, which had proclaimed that the NHS provided good value for money and high levels of satisfaction, and thus did not need 'major surgery'. Its recommendations had involved measures to strengthen and simplify management of the NHS, but no 'major surgery'. Prime Minister Margaret Thatcher, however, was not satisfied that the commission had gone far enough. In 1983 she commissioned another report to be conducted by four business leaders and chaired by Roy Griffiths of Sainsbury's. As a result, existing management teams were swept away and a system of 'general management' introduced, with the NHS Management Board (headed in the early days by Griffiths, who received a knighthood for his 'services to the National Health Service'[1] rather than to business) responsible for finances and policy.[2] It was intended to increase efficiency, but the funding crisis got worse.

In 1988 Margaret Thatcher was under great pressure over the NHS. The UK was at the time spending far less on health than the average country in the Organisation for Co-operation and Development (OECD), but the newspapers were filled with the story of Matthew Collier, a four-year-old boy who had been listed five times for hospital admission for heart surgery, and five times the admission was cancelled because there were no beds. His parents were taking the NHS to court. The Prime Minister was reported as saying that she would never again be held responsible for the NHS. Soon, in the course of a *Panorama* programme, she announced another review, taking her own ministers by surprise.

The resulting NHS and Community Care Act 1990 introduced two major changes.[3] One was the creation of the internal market, where health organisations were to buy services from one another. The other was GP fundholding. On the face of it, fundholding was an ingenious strategy for distancing government from responsibility for the delivery of clinical services. If the GPs were given the budgets, then they would become responsible for creating and managing waiting lists and for any rationing of health care. Given that successive MORI polls have showed doctors to be the most trusted of the professions (politicians the least trusted), this should have taken the pressure off the government, in particular the Prime Minister and the Secretary of State for Health, Kenneth Clarke. Central government could squeeze NHS overall spending, and the consequent shortfall in provision could be laid at the door of GPs. The tactic did not work. GP fundholding was optional and only covered part of the NHS's total spend. Despite powerful incentives, in the form of both sticks and carrots, only half the GPs had taken up fundholding in the first five years of the policy. And, of course, less than six months after the bill's enactment, John Major became Prime Minister.

In 1997 Labour was elected, and two years later Tony Blair's government abolished fundholding. They did not, however, drop the underlying principles put in place by Thatcher. Labour promoted so-called 'practice-based commissioning'. Though many GPs, including myself, who were ethically opposed to fundholding did approve of GPs being involved in the commissioning of services, it did not make sense to commission services at such a local level. Individual GPs could not see the overall picture of national health needs, even less the requirements for specialist and referral services. There wasn't the necessary expertise. The variation in demand from one practice to another, from one year to the next, made the allocation of even notional budgets unworkable. But the real sticking point was that the clinician looking after the patient should not, we felt, be holding the budget.[4]

Whilst Labour went quiet on the budgetary side of NHS management in the early years, they were far from inactive when it came to developing the market in health care. Increasingly, Labour favoured external competition over internal competition within the NHS. Private companies were brought in to provide everything from transport and information technology to primary care, hospital services and even capital development through the woefully inefficient and expensive Private Finance Initiative (PFI).[5] Initially, private sector providers were brought in only where it seemed that there was need for extra capacity to deal with a waiting list problem, or where it was difficult to recruit GPs. Soon, however, this fig leaf was dropped and commissioners were under pressure to give contracts to private companies, even where there was a perfectly acceptable local NHS service that had the support of local patients and the local council.

So Lansley's plans did not fill me with enthusiasm. There were others who saw the warning signs from the outset: a number of senior doctors and a few politicians, including two Liberal Democrat MPs: John Pugh, who represents Southport, and who was appointed to be the co-chair of the Liberal Democrat Parliamentary Committee for Health and Social Care, and Andrew George, who represents the West Cornwall and Scilly constituency of St Ives and who is the party's member on the Health Select Committee. Unfortunately, though, the medical professions and the public were slow to appreciate the very real threat to the NHS. What is more, some of the more sinister elements of Lansley's proposals did not become clear until the text of the Health and Social Care Bill was published the following year.

MOTIONS TO OPPOSE

For some years, I had been speaking out on the damaging changes to the NHS introduced by successive Tory and Labour governments. The Liberal Democrats constitutionally set party policy during formal debates at our national conferences. In 2008 I took an amendment to a health policy motion in order to draw attention to the damage being done by privatisation and fragmentation. It included the requirement that:

No further private sector procurement should be permitted unless it meets four criteria:

1. That the new service meets all NHS standards for quality, information and communication.
2. That the new service will provide the full range of services to the full range of patients that are being provided by the NHS service which it is intended to replace, or with which it is intended to compete.
3. That it can demonstrate that it is better value for money than the service it is replacing, or with which it is intended to compete.
4. That it can demonstrate that it will not destabilise local NHS facilities.

The amendment received overwhelming support.

By the time Lansley's White Paper was published, however, it was too late to submit an ordinary motion to the Liberal Democrats' 2010 autumn conference in Liverpool. Thankfully, I could still submit an emergency motion to the conference, and I did. When my motion was seen by Paul Burstow, at that time Junior Health Minister in the Coalition, he contacted me to try to arrange a meeting. The conference agenda had two slots for emergency motions, and the motions that would get an airing would be chosen by a ballot of delegates. Prior to the conference, my motion was expected to be allocated one of the slots. Yet the conference committee decided to allocate one of the emergency debates to an expression of concern and sympathy over the floods in Pakistan.[6] The other slot went to a motion calling for alternatives to Trident as part of the defence and security review.[7] After the conference, Burstow forgot that he wanted to meet me.

In January 2011 I submitted a motion for the spring party conference in Sheffield. Again I sought to point out that Lansley's proposals were incompatible with Liberal Democrat policy and would harm the delivery of health services to our constituents. Paul Burstow also submitted a motion. In it he denigrated the NHS with a series of false or misleading statistics and praised Lansley's vision of a new version of the NHS that could aspire to be among the best in the world, with reduced inequalities in services and more focus on patients, carers, clinicians and local authorities. Ironically Burstow claimed that this new version would involve less fragmentation of services. When I reported on the errors in his statistics, he rewrote the motion, drawing upon a different, but equally misleading, set of statistics.

Perhaps predictably, the conference committee chose Burstow's motion in preference to mine. However, I was told that they hoped I would put forward an amendment to it. That posed something of a dilemma, since the Liberal Democrat constitution does not allow 'wrecking amendments'. I could not, for example, insert the word 'not' into every sentence – though there was the temptation! I was, therefore, facing significant constraints on what I could insert or delete as part of my amendment. However, given that much of Burstow's motion carried on about 'motherhood and apple-pie', I had an opportunity. I could leave much of the motion unchanged and introduce many of the major concerns about the White Paper into the amendment, where they would be getting their first mention.

By now awareness of the White Paper had grown within the party, and we had ten times the support normally required for an amendment. Three local parties gave formal endorsement, and two senior Lib Dems, Evan Harris and Graham Winyard, who were also doctors, gave tireless support. Harris had been a member of the Shadow Cabinet until the 2010 general election. At one time he had served as the party's health spokesman. Winyard was chair of Winchester Liberal Democrats, but he also brought a background in public health and had served as deputy chief medical officer and medical director of the NHS.

During the run-up to the debate over the amendment, I asked Baroness Shirley Williams if she would sign on to support us. She replied that she did not want to give formal support, fearing that some members might support the amendment 'out of sentimental attachment to a veteran Lib Dem' and, presumably, not on the merits of our statement. The nobility of that stance was somewhat dulled when she delivered a passionate speech in favour of the amendment.

When it came time for the debate, every speech was in support of the amendment, and Burstow conceded graciously. In fact we managed to pass two amendments to Burstow's motion and deleted the lines that quoted misleading figures about the performance of the NHS in Britain. The media could be in no doubt whatsoever that the Liberal Democrat membership had given a thumbs down to Lansley.

As we Lib Dems were making our opposition vocal, even some Conservatives in the Coalition were expressing concern. Stephen Dorrell, who chaired the backbench Health Committee, regarded the structural reforms as a high risk politically – with the potential to damage the NHS at a time when it was facing enormous economic challenges due to the recession. Norman Tebbit, who had served in Thatcher's Cabinet and whose wife was severely injured in the bombing at the Grand Hotel, Brighton, during the party conference in 1984, was even more outspoken. He had seen at first hand how NHS services had been threatened when the private sector cherry-picked simpler orthopaedic work from the caseload of the specialist orthopaedic unit in Oxford.

With opposition mounting, Deputy Prime Minister and leader of the Liberal Democrats Nick Clegg agreed to the proposed 'listening pause' devised to push the health bill through Parliament. Interestingly, whereas Lansley promised to 'pause, listen and engage', the Prime Minister's spokesperson described the purpose of this unusual tactic as to 'pause, listen, engage and amend' the bill.

On 6 April 2011 the Coalition Government announced the formation of the NHS Future Forum. The forum had forty-five members. The chairman was Professor Steve Field, who until the previous November had been chairman of the Royal College of General Practitioners (RCGP) and had since worked with a number of groups on the implementation of the proposal for GP commissioning consortia. Field said that he had no hand in drafting Lansley's White Paper, but admitted that he liked it – he was 'absolutely behind' its principles.

The Future Forum was asked to gather feedback on four main themes, each handled by a separate working group:

1. Choice and Competition – chaired by Sir Stephen Bubb, chief executive of the Association of Chief Executives of Voluntary Organisations (Acevo).

2. Clinical Advice and Leadership – chaired by Dr Kathy McLean, medical director of NHS East Midlands.

3. Education and Training – chaired by Julie Moore, chief executive of University Hospitals Birmingham.

4. Patient and Public Involvement – chaired by Geoff Alltimes, chief executive of Hammersmith and Fulham Borough Council.

Acevo had been campaigning for a bigger role for the voluntary sector in public services and had been in touch with Andrew Lansley before the 'pause' to see what could be done to promote the idea of 'voluntary sector providers in the reforms'. This put Bubb's neutrality into question. John Pugh MP (Southport), pointed out that Bubb was also chair of the Trustees of the Adventure Capital Fund, which provides finance for 'third-sector' organisations. The fund says that the company 'expects a return on our investment – we hold our investees to account to provide us with results, both social and financial'.[8] At the time of Bubb's appointment to the Future Forum, he also had close contact with key lobbyists for several private sector companies that sell services to the NHS.

Bubb's report to Cameron's Cabinet was fulsome in its praise of competition, including competition from the private sector. According to his own account, posted on his internet site Bubb's Blog, he states his 'final plea to the Cabinet; not to be wimpy about competition'.[9]

Five of the forty-five members of the Future Forum were practising GPs. All of them had some previous connection to the reforms, either as outspoken supporters or as leaders of the pathfinder consortia being set up at that time. In January 2011 Charles Alessi, a GP in Kingston upon Thames, wrote an article in the *Sun* entitled 'NHS shake-up will be better for docs, better for patients',[10] and appeared on television praising the reforms. By February of the next year he had changed his view and was telling the *Guardian* that GPs would be 'suffocated rather than liberated' by the changes.[11] In May his Surrey practice was back in the paper's pages when it was found to have removed forty-eight elderly and disabled patients from the practice list, 'predominantly for financial reasons'.[12] This sort of discrimination against patients with heavy care demands (and high costs to the practice) is common in many market-driven health services, and has long been a point of controversy in American health maintenance organisations (HMOs), including those that receive money from the government-sponsored Medicare programme.[13]

In reality there was neither a pause, nor much listening, from the Future Forum. At panel meetings there was more evidence of talking than listening. During this period Graham Winyard and I offered to meet Nick Clegg to explain our concerns. Between us we had extensive experience of the NHS. My background is in general practice, health information and IT, and I had managed hospitals and community services locally, and as I've already shared, Graham's background was in public health and NHS management at the highest level. Nevertheless, at no time did Clegg agree to see us. One might be forgiven for thinking that he did not want to be told about the problems with the bill.

The government's response to the Future Forum was to announce some modifications to the bill, but none were fundamental. And the government had prepared its response even before the panel had reported. On 7 June Bubb wrote on his blog that: 'Just as I was signing off on our Panel's report on "Delivering real choice" I get sent a copy of the PM speech announcing he is accepting many of our key recommendations (although we haven't actually given him the report yet!)'.[14]

As already noted, GPs would be reorganised into clinical commissioning groups (CCGs), which would have a hospital doctor as well as lay members, and would be required to consult clinical networks and some new bodies called 'clinical senates'. Foundation trusts were to have public board meetings. The health and well-being committees of local authorities would have the right to refer any commissioning plans with the agreed-upon health and well-being strategy to the NHS Commissioning Board (NHSCB). We were told that the CCGs, NHSCB and the regulator Monitor would together promote integrated care, but there was no hint as to how this was to be done, and it seemed to stand as a lower priority than promoting choice and competition. We were also told that new safeguards against price competition, cherry-picking and privatisation would be put in place, though we were not told what these would be, or how Monitor or the NHSCB would deliver any such safeguards.

The post-pause bill contained a few ideas for improving care. A new body called Health Education England was to 'ensure a safe and robust transition for the education and training system'. No clue was offered as to how this would be delivered, or whether it would have any influence on the commissioning process to ensure that trainees would have access to clinical material they need to learn. Another new body, Public Health England, was to co-ordinate public health, which was being devolved to local authorities. CCGs, NHSCB and Public Health England would, we were told, promote research, but no detail was given as to how this would happen or how this initiative would sit alongside the other duties and priorities of these bodies.

TOO LITTLE, TOO LATE

On 10 June 2011 Nick Clegg spent an hour and a half on the phone with Evan Harris, Graham Winyard and me, explaining the concessions that he had negotiated with the Prime Minister. On the face of it, the changes seemed encouraging. He claimed to have delivered on the majority of the points we had made in the spring party conference, though there were some he admitted he had been unable to deliver. Even at the time, I realised that there were significant unresolved issues – most importantly issues relating to conflict of interest, fragmentation of care, the

challenge of ensuring collaboration between competing providers, the destabilising of established services by competition from
new providers, and the need for teaching, training and education.

Just a few days later, on 14 June, David Cameron made a
speech at Guy's Hospital, London, in which he seemed to pull
back from many of the assurances that had been given to us by
Clegg. On 20 June, the government published its formal response
to the 'listening' pause and it became apparent that very little of
substance had been conceded by the Tories.

One of our key concerns had been the desire of the Secretary
of State to absolve himself of the responsibility for the provision of health care in England. Clegg had assured us that the
clause referring to the Secretary of State's responsibilities had
been reinstated 'word for word' from the previous NHS acts. It
turned out that he was referring to a completely different clause,
one that referred only to a 'duty to promote' health care. Indeed,
the government's response on the duty of the Secretary of State
read: 'we'll make clear in the Bill that Ministers are responsible
for the NHS overall – the original duty to promote a comprehensive health service will remain'.[15] But this referred only to Clause
S1(1) of the previous acts, which required the Secretary of State
to promote a service. Clause S3(1), which required the Secretary
of State to provide or secure provision of services, had been
removed. In addition, the 'amended' bill granted a brand-new level
of autonomy to organisations within the NHS structure and, in
the process, the Secretary of State lost the ability to direct either
providers or commissioners.

Over the following months, Andrew Lansley's staff at the
Department of Health (DoH) seemed determined to remove
all references to the word 'provide' in the health bill. The NHS
would, if the bill was passed, gradually cease to be a *provider* of
health care and shift to being a commissioner of health care from

independent providers, many of which, of course, would likely come from the private sector.

The other matter of deep concern was the retention of competition as a key objective in the reform proposals. In Clegg's conversation with us he had made much of the fact that Monitor would no longer have as a prime responsibility the promotion of competition. It would go back to a purer role, 'to protect and promote the interests of patients'. It turned out, however, that the responsibility for promoting competition had simply been moved to the NHS Commissioning Board, and many of the references to competition in the bill had been rephrased to use the word 'choice'.

Few things irritated me more over the next few months than the repeated claim from the Liberal Democrats' leadership that we had addressed nearly all of the objections we had raised in Sheffield, and that it was time for troublemakers like me, Harris and Winyard to stop complaining and claim success. Even Clegg conceded that he had not delivered on all the points made in the Sheffield amendment. In addition, as I repeatedly pointed out during the debates, there had been severe constraints as to what I could include in the amendment to Burstow's motion. What is more, the Sheffield debate had been on Lansley's White Paper, not on the health bill that was presented to Parliament.

Through August and early September 2011 my concerns grew. During the committee stage Andrew George proposed a raft of additional amendments to handle some of the unresolved issues. These were thrown out by the Tory majority. The only course left was to go back to the Lib Dem membership at the autumn 2011 party conference in Birmingham.

We prepared a motion. Though it had a record number of backers, it was rejected by the conference committee.[16] We therefore submitted an emergency motion with yet another new record number of supporters for bringing the issue to the membership. Nevertheless, the conference committee refused to put it on the list of motions to go into the ballot for members to decide. Instead they scheduled an anodyne discussion item on the health bill, with no resolution and no vote. A motion on responding to that summer's riots had won the committee's emergency slot.

At the conference we proposed the suspension of standing orders so that the party membership in attendance could choose whether to debate our motion. The vote took place early in the morning on the first day of the conference, Saturday, 17 September, at a time when the conference hall is usually pretty empty and rather routine reports are taken. We had the support of the majority of those attending, but the suspension of standing orders requires the support of two-thirds of those voting, and we lost by a count of 235 in favour to 183 against.[17] How strange it was to see all those MPs and peers leaving the hall after the vote. We were forced to the conclusion that the parliamentarians had been whipped to turn out against us.

Later in the autumn the Health and Social Care Bill returned to the House of Lords for further scrutiny. Though a thousand amendments had been made to it, many were trivial, and even those that looked substantive proved to be somewhat illusory. Lansley declared himself happy that nothing of the central thrust of his proposals had been removed. Throughout this period Graham Winyard and I continued to attend the Liberal Democrat Parliamentary Health Committee to ensure that none of the committee members could be in doubt about the continuing problems with Lansley's bill. Despite all the evidence to the contrary, there were still many who felt that the bill could be amended sufficiently to prevent serious damage to the NHS.

THE LAST EMERGENCY

Throughout the winter more minor amendments were passed in the Lords, and things came to a head in the spring. The parliamentary session was scheduled to end on 1 May 2012, and the government clearly wanted the bill to get through all the necessary stages towards passing by the end of March. In a final bid to carry the day, Clegg persuaded Shirley Williams to join him in writing a letter that stated major and significant changes had been realised in the bill and promising that yet more would be sought. It was sent first to MPs and peers, then to every member of the party. Many of the claims in Clegg and Williams's letter were wrong, spurious or irrelevant.[18] Consider these lines from it, against the reality:

1.   *'competition could only be on quality and not on price'*: Under procurement law one of two procedures must be used whenever public sector procurement of health services is carried out through competitive tendering. One is based purely on cost, and the other combines cost and quality.

2.   *'the Secretary of State will remain responsible and accountable for a comprehensive health service'*: As mentioned, this clause was reworded several times but, with every version, the Secretary of State's role in NHS accountability was effectively reduced. The government steadfastly refused to retain the wording from sections 2 and 3 of the 2006 NHS act. Under all previous NHS acts it was the Secretary of State who

determined what services it was appropriate for patients to receive from the NHS; in future it will be up to each CCG to determine what is appropriate, and the Secretary of State does not have direct oversight of the CCGs. In addition, providers in a free market cannot be forced to offer a comprehensive service, and based on the law of the market and logic, they will provide only what they believe can be profitable.

3.   *'arrangements have been put in place to make the UK a world leader in medical research'*: Thus far, the primary area where this research initiative has been specified is in the collecting and sharing of data with the pharmaceutical industry for development of novel therapies. This will be an expensive proposition for the NHS and a profitable one for the private companies, which will be able to receive patent protection for any new drugs they develop. However, there is no mechanism for meeting the NHS costs for collecting and sharing this potentially rich mine of information.

4.   *'raise the status and protect the independence of the Public Health service'*: Public health experts disagree with claims that they have been protected or given more influence, with many reporting that the public health service has been fragmented by the Health and Social Care Act. Some public health experts have stayed with the NHS, but some have been moved to local authorities (where they receive no dedicated funding for their efforts) and some have moved

to the private sector. The voice of public health specialists has been weakened as a result.

5. *'all profits from the treatment of private patients in Foundation Trust hospitals must benefit the NHS'*: Foundation trust hospitals have not-for-profit status, so to do anything else would have been illegal.

6. *'safeguards to stop private providers "cherry picking"'*: Cherry-picking has not been eliminated. Providers are required only to set out the eligibility criteria determining which patients they are prepared to treat. This does not prevent cherry-picking, it merely *documents* it. As providers cannot be forced to take on patients they are not competent or qualified to treat (under 'Any Qualified Provider' rules), it will be impossible to eliminate selection of patients by providers.

7. *'decisions about patient services and taxpayers' money must be made in an open, transparent and accountable way'*: Private sector providers have no obligation to supply nor even collect information about their patient numbers or outcomes. Where the public sector has this information about a private provider, the private company can block its publication, even when requests are made under the Freedom of Information Act, by claiming the 'commercial sensitivity' of the data. Indeed, neither private sector providers nor private companies supporting the commissioning process are covered by the Freedom of Information Act – only

government bodies are held to this level of public scrutiny.

8. *'there will be real democratic accountability in the NHS through new Health and Wellbeing Boards'*: Health and Wellbeing boards have a minimal elected element, and no right to do more than write letters of complaint. Provisions in the bill for local Healthwatch units were never strong. Healthwatch England, which is now being set up, lacks any effective means of influencing events. More troubling is the fact that Healthwatch England will be a subunit of the Care Quality Commission (CQC), and many Healthwatch complaints about care will likely implicate the CQC for failing to address the problem – provoking a conflict of interest for the CQC if Healthwatch investigates the complaints.

In order for an emergency motion to be put to party conference, it is necessary that something significant must have happened after the closing date for normal motions. We believed that the Clegg/Williams letter was such a development. In addition, the government had defied orders from the information commissioner to publish the Risk Register relating to the health bill and the consequences of a reorganisation of the NHS under the bill's provisions.[19] Moreover, almost all the medical royal colleges had now moved to a position where they were asking for the bill to be dropped completely. The Prime Minister had called an emergency summit, sensing the shift in mood. We felt that we had full justification for an emergency motion demanding that the health bill be withdrawn or defeated.

We arrived at Gateshead for the spring party conference on 9 March 2012 to discover that our emergency motion was one of four competing for a single slot on the agenda. There were also motions on Justice and on Syria, as well as one bizarrely entitled 'Protecting our NHS: the Shirley Williams motion'. Could this have been the same Shirley Williams who was reluctant to allow her name to appear on a list of those supporting our Sheffield amendment in case people voted 'out of sentimental attachment to the old lady'? The Williams motion said, more or less, that we have made a lot of changes to the health bill, haven't we done well? Now it is time to pass it. (The exact words were 'achieved significant changes' and 'taking the lead from the motion passed at Spring Conference 2011 … have worked successfully'.[20]) I for one could not see how that qualified as an emergency motion.

There was heavy lobbying for the two rival motions, ours and the Williams motion. We were bound by conference rules to stay outside the building for our lobbying, but there were demonstrations outside the Sage conference centre and we distributed leaflets to delegates as they arrived. The party leader's team also distributed leaflets outside, but in addition put leaflets in every delegate's pack and on every chair in advance of a ministerial question session.

In the ballot our motion won the greatest number of first preference votes, but when second preference votes were counted, as required, the Williams motion was selected for debate. We believe that the leader's office was hoping to avoid any real debate about the NHS, and therefore instructed MPs and peers to put the Syria motion first and the Williams motion second. Undaunted, we pushed to delete the crucial lines from the Williams motion that would have said: 'Conference Calls on Liberal Democrat peers to support the Third Reading of the Bill provided such further amendments are achieved.' We were successful.

Once again the media could be in no doubt about the opposition to the bill within the Lib Dem membership. The BBC's Norman Smith tweeted, 'Major setback for Nick Clegg at Lib Dem conference as party members vote by crushing majority 314-217 NOT to back health bill.'

Nine days later, on 20 March 2012, the Health and Social Care Act became law.

VESTED INTERESTS

I have thus far confined myself to reporting what happened. I shall now explore briefly some of the possible 'whys' underlying this chain of events, which requires going beyond my main focus on the Liberal Democrat party's actions in 2011–13.

As detailed in chapter 2, Labour were slow to criticise the bill when it was introduced to Parliament. This may have come down to the party's own record of promoting private providers and market competition in the NHS. Although the Thatcher government had made inroads towards bringing the market to bear on the NHS, there was far more privatisation undertaken in the Blair and Brown governments. Under Thatcher, cleaning contracts were put out to tender; under Blair and Brown, private providers were given contracts for radiology, surgery and transport services, and for the creation of walk-in centres and GP services. The walk-in centres as well as NHS Direct were set up with the supposed aim of offering increased choice to patients, but in fact these initiatives weakened the concept of a GP as the patient's single entry point to health services. While there clearly are some places where GP services are not adequate to serve patient needs, introducing these parallel services should never have been regarded as an efficient way to address such deficiencies.

But this was just the beginning. Step by step, the relationship between patient and GP was made more tenuous. After NHS Direct was introduced, the government negotiated a new contract with the GP Committee of the British Medical Association (BMA). There was a new emphasis on targets and outcomes, and for the first time GPs could give up the commitment to twenty-four-hour care in return for a reduction in remuneration. The contract was then further altered so that patients no longer were registered with an individual GP but with an entire practice.

Two alternative ways of employing GPs were then introduced.[21] Alternative Provider Medical Services (APMS) contracts were initially promoted as a way of providing primary care in localities where it was otherwise impossible to recruit doctors. That pretence was soon dropped and private providers were introduced in the north of England, in Derbyshire and in London, where there were no recruitment problems. Many of these contracts were won by UnitedHealth Group, who had only recently paid millions of dollars in the US to settle claims related to alleged defrauding of patients, doctors and insurers.[22] Gradually patients were losing their unique personal relationship with their doctor. Patients were to become parts of an anonymous client base that could be bought and sold by companies in takeover bids.

In the last four years of the Labour Government there was a rapid rise in the number of NHS patients being treated by private providers.[23] For example, 17 per cent of NHS hernia and hip replacement operations were bought from private providers. It appears that little thought was given at the time to how this might destabilise the NHS and undermine the training of doctors. At one point, for instance, all of the cataract operations in the Oxford area were going to a private provider, which was paid to take on the work. At the same time, the local NHS hospital was expected to be training the next generation of surgeons in eye operations, despite having no cataract patients for them to work with.

In 2006 the DoH advertised for multinational firms to take over the purchasing of health care with budgets of up to £64 billion.[24] They also introduced a half-way stage whereby external firms could do some of the work of commissioning services as well as providing them.[25] By 2010 there were thirteen firms approved to take on this work, including Aetna UK, AXA PPP Healthcare, Bupa Health Dialog, CHKS (with the slogan 'Insight for better healthcare'), Dr Foster Intelligence (with the slogan 'Using the power of information to provide better services'), Humana Europe, KPMG, McKesson Corporation, McKinsey & Company, Navigant Consulting, Tribal Health Commissioning, UnitedHealth Group and WG Consulting. It has been reported elsewhere in this book that by this time Labour had plans to hand the whole of commissioning over to external management consultants, without even the fig-leaf pretence of GP involvement that Lansley chose to include in his reforms in order to gain Coalition buy-in.

Labour politicians also made full use of the revolving door between industry and government. Alan Milburn and Patricia Hewitt are among the ten previous health ministers who have taken lucrative consultancies with private health care companies.[26] In January 2009 Tony Blair's health adviser Simon Stevens became executive vice president of UnitedHealth Group, responsible for that company's global expansion as president of Global Health.[27]

Labour has been just as involved as the Tories in the use of private management consultants to develop policy and advise on implementation. In 2009–10 the DoH paid more than £26 million to private consultancies, with the American firm McKinsey & Company heading the pack.[28]

LOSS OF LEADERSHIP

While the actions of the Liberal Democrats have been enumerated above, there are also two key questions about the motivations that framed them, namely: 1) Why did Nick Clegg ignore the advice he was offered? 2) What was Shirley Williams up to?

To answer these questions, and to consider the significance of the coalition between the Lib Dems and the Tories, it is important to remember that every political party is a coalition within itself. The culture within the Liberal Democrat Party has two main strands. First, the nineteenth-century liberalism of Gladstone, of free trade, small government, freedom of the individual and equality of opportunity. Then there is the twentieth-century liberalism of Lloyd George and William Beveridge, of social liberalism that emphasises fairness and a caring, sharing society that may well allow for the state to take a larger role in people's lives. In my experience, these two strands do not comprise rival groups, but are present to a greater or lesser extent in all members. Nevertheless, there are some who embrace the free market, small government aspect of liberalism with rather more zeal than others. For instance, in 2004 David Laws advocated the replacement of the NHS with a National Health Insurance Scheme. In 2005 Nick Clegg said, in an interview with the *Independent*, 'I think breaking up the NHS is exactly what you do need to do to make it a more responsive service.'[29]

With that historical legacy backing up the groupthink endemic in Westminster, one could imagine that Nick Clegg made up his mind in favour of Lansley's bill. In that case, perhaps the last thing he would welcome was contrary opinion from his backbenchers and party members, let alone confusion around the public message. Little wonder he had not wished to meet with Graham Winyard and me. But, of course, we were not alone in criticising the reform package. People working in every branch of the NHS, as well as academics, health economists and public health experts were saying that Lansley's plans were costly, cumbersome and damaging to the care of patients. It would be bad for the NHS, bad for patients and bad for the health of Britain, but it seems that our party leader did not wish to hear the evidence.

To committed activists like myself, Shirley Williams's position was, and continues to be, more confusing and more confused. As described in chapter 3, in March 2011, after Williams declined to sign up to our amendment, she went on to speak passionately in its favour. She wrote that Lansley's reforms would 'dismember' the service through this 'untried and disruptive' reorganisation.[30] In September she signed up to our emergency motion and wrote that 'this flawed bill threatens the very future of the NHS'.[31] Yet only five months later she joined Clegg in signing a letter to their fellow Lib Dem MPs and peers that made claims and reassurances on the subjects of the duties of the Secretary of State; the capacity for Britain to lead the world in medical research; on the potential for cherry-picking of profitable services away from the NHS; the focus of the introduction of competition on price; the use of democratic channels to ensure health care accountability; and an insistence that the plan would not allow a takeover of the system by private health care providers. Finally, and most surprisingly, she allowed her name to be put to a motion endorsing the health bill.

Despite several conversations with Shirley Williams, I cannot claim to understand fully her fluctuating position. It was clear from the outset that she did not take on board all my concerns with Lansley's proposals. I suspect that she did not understand some of the issues I was raising about the linkage between various clinical practices caring for the same patient, or the complexity of co-ordinated medical care. It may be obvious that if a consultant obstetrician performs a Caesarian section the result will be the birth of a baby who may need the attention of a paediatrician. The fact that the consultant obstetrician is also a gynaecologist who treats patients with cancer means that some of that doctor's patients will need access to radiotherapy services – it's not enough to link obstetricians with paediatricians; they need to be linked with a large range of other consultants. Similarly, orthopaedic surgeons may conduct pre-planned operations on hips, knees, backs and hands, but they also attend to the victims of major accident injuries who arrive at an A&E and need attention immediately, regardless of the surgeries already scheduled for the day. For any one part of a hospital service to operate efficiently, it needs to be closely linked to many other departments. This is particularly plain in the case of older patients who often suffer from a multitude of illnesses and in whom elective surgery may require the support of many different specialists, whose attention and treatment needs to be co-ordinated with rehabilitation and social services afterwards.

It also worried me that Lansley's proposals had not – and could not, in practice – ensure that there would be no cherry-picking of profitable services by private health care providers, a promise that has since been quietly dropped. The ever-shifting position of the DoH on this question would suggest that officials there are aware of the practical limitations involved.

The DoH was adamant throughout the negotiations that the word 'provide' was taboo with respect to the role of the Secretary of State. The NHS acts of 1946, 1966, 1977 and 2006 all committed the Secretary of State for Health to promote a comprehensive health service; provide or secure provision of such services (listed in the acts themselves); and ensure that the health service should be free of charge except as expressly provided by legislation. Only the first of these three principles survived in the Health and Social Care Act 2012, and subsequent clauses have limited significantly the powers of the Secretary of State. This issue has been the subject of intensive legal scrutiny, and Shirley Williams herself took legal advice on it in July 2011. She was advised that the new health bill put no legal obligation on the Secretary of State to provide and secure a comprehensive NHS. It would be interesting to know whether her change of position in February 2012 was informed by further legal advice or just by rhetoric and repeated assertions from Clegg's office.

Some have suggested that Shirley Williams was bullied into changing her position. I myself rather doubt that she could be so easily bullied. She is, however, an experienced and successful politician, and experienced and successful politicians may sometimes decide to take a pragmatic view. Whereas the idealist who wins some concessions but doesn't win the whole case will say, 'If only we had started earlier. If only we had had more support. If only ...', the pragmatist determines the point at which all the concessions that might be won have been won and declares that outcome to be both satisfactory and successful.

REVOLVING DOORS

There was a scandal when Channel 4 exposed a number of senior MPs selling themselves like a taxi cab plying for trade.[32] But the revolving door is often used among MPs and ministers: special advisers in particular come and go – one minute they are giving advice to ministers, the next working for the very companies who stand to benefit from decisions based on that advice.

As already recounted, management consultancies McKinsey, PA Consulting Group, KPMG, PricewaterhouseCoopers, Ernst & Young and Deloitte Touche Tohmatsu Ltd have had major contracts with the DoH. These firms also work for private health care companies that are already benefiting from the government's NHS reforms. But if one looks more widely, scanning the financial links between health care companies and politicians, it becomes obvious that the contagion is still worse. Seventy MPs and 142 peers have a vested interest in the promotion of private health care.[33] If members of a local council had a similar interest in a matter of policy, they would be barred from voting on any relevant regulations or measures. In Parliament, however, MPs and peers are allowed to vote regardless of their interests, and most of them did in the case of Lansley's health bill.

The issue of vested interest is still highly relevant, these many months after the passing of the Health and Social Care Act. The body charged with seeing fair play in the operation of the commercial market in health care, the Co-operation and Competition Panel (CCP), is led by Patrick Carter, Baron Carter of Coles, who founded Westminster Health Care, a private nursing home company that is now part of Barchester Healthcare, now the fourth largest private health care provider in the UK. A Labour peer, Lord Carter, is chairman of McKesson Information Solutions Ltd, a subsidiary of the American conglomerate McKesson Corporation that sells IT to the NHS. In an interview with the *Guardian*, Clare Gerada of the Royal College of General Practitioners said: 'He cannot have any credibility when he is also heading a company with such huge interests in the very contracts his organisation is meant to police. GPs are being minutely scrutinised for possible conflicts of interest ... if we are going to have to have transparency, it has to apply throughout the system.'[34] McKesson is not his only area of interest in the private health care market. He is also chair of, adviser to and shareholder in a number of other companies with interests in health care, such as the private equity investment firm Warburg Pincus International and the Bermuda-based Primary Group Ltd.

In such an incestuous world it is perhaps surprising that anyone in the Westminster bubble has managed to remain uncontaminated by the influence of the free marketeers. Caught between lobbyists and international corporations, the NHS had little chance – or rather, it will have little chance unless we take steps, before it is too late – to reverse its sale and destruction.

6

HIDDEN IN PLAIN SIGHT

Oliver Huitson

It is fascinating to note here how one of the BBC's senior correspondents had thoroughly internalised the Downing Street constructed narrative of events... [they] did not merely present the Downing Street line very faithfully – it was almost as if [the Prime Minister] was speaking.

Peter Oborne, *The Triumph of the Political Class*

Damaging scoops and servile blandishments, expert analysis and lobbyist-led churnalism, craven fawning from the BBC alongside damning exposés from the *Daily Mail* – this is the story of the media's representation of the Health and Social Care Act 2012. Throughout it all, with a few notable exceptions, the media machine appeared to be highly vulnerable to influences coming from Downing Street and the health care industry. The debates around this massive piece of legislation were often reduced to trivia and misrepresentation, including the mantra that unions, sometimes depicted as the sole 'vested interests' in the fight, were merely pushing back against 'modernisation'; the playground game of 'Labour did it first' as a means of shirking responsibility for passing the bill; the chant-like declaration that the reforms would empower GPs; and haggling over whether meaningless sops to the Lib Dems were victories for David Cameron or Nick Clegg. While the debate raged, Cameron could assure his target audience – which surely wasn't the general public, given the polling at the time – that the 'fundamentals' of the bill remained in place.

But what were the 'fundamentals' of the bill, and what did the public know about them? How did the media stand up when it came to its role? As Lord Justice Leveson has put it: 'The press provides an essential check on all aspects of public life. That is why any failure within the media affects all of us.'[1] Did the media adequately report, let alone investigate, the origins of the health bill, its implications, the forces driving it, the government's claims about its repercussions and, ultimately, who stood to benefit? These were not unreasonable questions, and it was the job of the media to provide answers, to share information about how a government policy affects all of us – indeed, our very health.

MANDATE FROM A VACUUM

Before the 2010 general election David Cameron had assured the public that there would be 'no more top-down reorganisations of the NHS'. Once Health Secretary Andrew Lansley's White Paper was released, however, this line was difficult to maintain. Cameron, realising the strength of opposition to the health reforms, tried to distance himself with talk of his 'surprise' at how far they went. Surprises 'visible from space' (as David Nicholson called them[2]) might be welcome at a children's birthday party, but not where the nation's health is concerned. Though the public certainly were surprised, David Cameron appears to have been perhaps economical with the truth. According to a Conservative special adviser, quoted in Nicholas Timmins's *Never Again?*: 'all those things [in the bill] were cleared by a policy board chaired by Cameron. So the idea that Cameron didn't know what was in it … He and Oliver Letwin helped write the Green Papers.'[3] Given the reports of Cameron's direct involvement, it appears that the public were intentionally deceived about the extent of the reforms – and about the fact that the Tories' vision for the NHS would involve major reorganisations.

This alone should have been a major scandal, reported across the media. Critics of the bill repeatedly and vociferously brought up the fact that the NHS would be undergoing a major reorganisation, from the bill's announcement right up to its passage into law, despite lack of popular mandate for such a move. Some press outlets raised multiple times the broken pledge and the issue of democratic mandate, though these rarely ran to more than a passing note, and never to the point of questioning the legitimacy of what was happening. On the BBC's *This Week* programme, Michael Portillo admitted, astonishingly, '[the Tories] didn't believe they could win an election if they told you what they were going to do'. Yet concerns over the health bill's democratic mandate were mentioned only twice by the BBC in their online news and analysis in the nearly two years of debate. For some reason, they did not deem it an issue worth exploring.

If Lansley's bill did not have a mandate from either the general public or the medical professions, who exactly was driving it forward? It was surely the role of the media to ask this question, and its corollary – who stood to benefit from the bill's enactment? Yet time and again in the drafting and cheerleading of the bill, the role of the private health care industry was ignored, distorted, even at times hidden.

THE SILENT ROLE OF THE PRIVATE SECTOR

In general Channel 4's coverage of the health bill was exemplary. They probed, they questioned, they dug and they frequently exposed the bill for what it was. For instance, on 2 March 2011 Channel 4 broke an enlightening story, based on a 'leaked document', on what 'GP commissioning' might look like in practice.[4] In the memo shared by Channel 4, a private health firm, Integrated Health Partners (IHP), proposed to set up a company to run commissioning on behalf of GPs, in return giving those GPs a share of profits on the services delivered. According to Channel 4, IHP founder Oliver Bernath, an ex-McKinsey man, planned to float the company on the stock exchange within five years. The *Guardian*[5] and the *Daily Mail*[6] ran with the story, yet it was never mentioned by the BBC or the rest of the press. Here was a well-connected health care firm openly gearing up for a for-profit health service, yet the majority of the media fell silent.

In October 2010, a few months after the publication of Lansley's White Paper, Mark Britnell, head of health for KPMG, the 'big four' accountancy firm that makes considerable profits from outsourced and privatised health care services, described how the NHS would be shown 'no mercy' and would become a 'state insurance provider, not a state deliverer'.[7] Britnell had worked closely with the Labour Government and was a former head of commissioning for the NHS. But his comments, reported by the *Guardian*, were not uncovered until 14 May 2011 in the middle of the 'listening' pause. The story emerged after word came that Britnell was invited to join David Cameron's 'kitchen cabinet' to advise on the NHS 'reforms'. This was a man at the top of Westminster health circles describing the coming demise of the NHS and yet the BBC did not mention the story for another four days after it broke. When the BBC did finally deign to do so, Britnell was raised only in passing to explain a quote from Nick Clegg, in which he reportedly told his fellow Liberal Democrats: 'People get confused when one day they hear politicians declare how much they love the NHS and the next they hear people describing themselves as government advisers saying that reform is a huge opportunity for big profits for health care corporations.'[8] Britnell's comments apparently didn't count as a story in their own right, however, and they were not mentioned again by the BBC. In contrast, the *Guardian*, *Mirror* and *Daily Mail*[9] wrote full articles on the issue (and reprised their coverage in March 2013 as Britnell's name was bandied about as a replacement for Sir David Nicholson as head of the NHS[10]).

On 12 February 2012 the *Mail on Sunday* ran a major scoop involving the global consultancy McKinsey & Company, which has been involved in some way – often with some significant remuneration – in events ranging from the privatisation of British Rail to the fiasco over replacing the UK's aircraft carriers (with the Enron scandal in between).[11] The story concerned Monitor, the 'independent' regulator of the new health market, which will promote competition through its statutory duty to 'prevent *anti*-competitive behaviour'. Its chair is David Bennett – ex-McKinsey. He leads a board and management team dominated by former McKinsey and KPMG executives. The *Mail on Sunday*'s scoop not only covered some of these links, but showed that Bennett had received over £6,000 of hospitality from his old firm, McKinsey, during a trip to New York, 'where he stayed at a five-star hotel and attended a lavish banquet, all paid for by McKinsey', despite what appeared to be a clear conflict of interest in his new role at Monitor.

Even more alarming, however, the newspaper revealed that: 'Many of the bill's proposals were drawn up by McKinsey and included in the legislation wholesale. One document says McKinsey has used its privileged access to "share information" with its corporate clients – which include the world's biggest private hospital firms – who are now set to bid for health service work … The company is already benefiting from contracts worth undisclosed millions with GPs arising from the bill. It has earned at least £13.8 million from Government health policy since the Coalition took office – and the bill opens up most of the current £106 billion NHS budget to the private sector, with much of it likely to go to McKinsey clients.' (Interestingly, in November 2010 McKinsey had predicted that UK health care could be a '£200bn industry by 2030' in a report that got a splash in the *Telegraph*, including the consultancy's action point 5: 'Unleash the growth potential of education and health'.[12])

The *Mail on Sunday*'s McKinsey report came while the Lords were debating the exact language of the Health and Social Care Bill. Those standing to make substantial profits if the health bill was passed seemed to have had a significant role in shaping it. This was a major story, a scoop to be chased, investigated and developed – except that it wasn't. Two days later, the BBC gave the revelations just 120 words – the equivalent of a Post-it note – in passing at the bottom of an article about Nick Clegg's defence of Andrew Lansley. Of those 120 words, over half constituted a government rebuttal from Health Minister Earl Howe.[13] The BBC failed to explain that Bennett and other senior Monitor staff were ex-McKinsey, or that McKinsey staff had actually written sections of the bill themselves – only stating that 'senior staff at the NHS body Monitor … had been entertained at the company's expense'. The *Mail on Sunday* article received no mention at all from the rest of the press, or even Channel 4, the lone exception being found in the pages of the *Guardian*.

Shortly after the bill passed into law, the conflicts of interest that might be unleashed by it were starkly revealed through research from False Economy, an anti-austerity site supported by the Trades Union Congress.[14] False Economy reported that in its survey of twenty-two clinical commissioning groups (CCGs), at least half – and sometimes all – of the GPs named to the board had a personal financial interest in health care firms. This finding brought into sharp focus what many had been warning: there would be enormous potential for conflicts of interest in handing billions of pounds to CCGs whose members had financial ties to the health industry outside the NHS. Of course it should have been plain from the outset that doctors are neither accountants nor purchasers. They have full-time roles in their area of expertise: medicine. So who else would be running the CCGs day to day? And as Dr Kambiz Boomla pointed out in the *Mirror* in 2010, few had the time for these extra responsibilities: 'GPs will not have time to do the extra work that these proposals will task them with … They will have to outsource the work to managers … For one, it could lead to a situation where private sector companies that advise or take over a GP consortium will then be placing contracts with sister companies. The provider and commissioner would be in business together – this is a huge conflict of interest.'[15]

The potential for conflicts of interest involving both GPs and private sector commissioners should have been central to any critical examination of the bill; however, in much of the media it was rarely touched upon, and the inevitability of private firms becoming involved in commissioning was frequently ignored. The notion that GPs would be the primary 'commissioners' dominated media descriptions of the bill. A Channel 4 report dated 21 November 2011 is noteworthy for the clarity with which it explained the emerging health market, and how 'GP commissioning' would function in reality: 'GPs say they have firm evidence now that the government is planning to privatise the National Health Service as part of its reforms … In a document seen by Channel 4 News, plans are laid out for how services will be bought for patients ... Richard Vautrey, deputy chair of the *British Medical Association*'s (BMA) GP committee, said that the document was quite explicit in suggesting that the government was going to create a market for private companies to come in and take over these services ...'[16] As Jonathan Tomlinson, an east London GP, explained to Channel 4, the scale of private involvement would be so large 'as to include absolutely everything that commissioning involves'. Yet it appears that only the *Guardian* and the *Telegraph* mentioned the story. The rest of the media, including the BBC, ignored it.

It was in this near vacuum of information that the health bill was publicly debated.

THE TIE THAT BINDS

Power, money and influence were often entirely absent from news coverage about the health bill, yet each of these ingredients in policymaking were cited countless times a day by members of the public in the online comment sections provided by media outlets. Health Secretary Andrew Lansley, for instance, was known to have been personally bankrolled by John Nash, chairman of Care UK, a health firm that stood to make considerable profits from the reforms, according to a January 2010 report in the *Telegraph*.[17] By 2010, the firm was generating 96 per cent of its £400 million business from the NHS, and Nash had donated £21,000 to Lansley's personal office in November 2009. Nash was also founder of Sovereign Capital, which owns a number of firms in the health care industry, and was given a peerage and a job as Schools Minister in January 2013 (his other business interests include sponsoring academy schools).[18] The story of Nash's donation was covered in full by the *Guardian*, *Mirror* and Channel 4 and received fleeting notice in the *Independent* and *Daily Mail*, yet it was never once mentioned by the BBC or the *Sun*. The *Telegraph* appears to have decided that the story – to which it had given a whole article when it broke – merited just a single paragraph in the two years the bill was being debated, in a story on Lansley's wife, Sally Low.[19] The consultancy she founded, Low Associates, boasted on its website of its ability to 'make the link between the public and private sectors' and also claimed to have 'set up a debate between a Minister and his shadow, which really captured the media's attention', as reported in the *Daily Mail*.[20] The BBC never covered the story.

In January 2011 the *Mirror* reported that the Tories had received over £750,000 from donors with major health care interests since David Cameron assumed leadership of the party in 2005.[21] Among the *Telegraph*, *Independent*, *Daily Mail*, *Sun* and the BBC, not one of them mentioned the donations. The extent of Conservative backing from the health care industry was never raised, despite Parliament's frequent scandals surrounding the influence and rewards that such donations tend to generate. In the case of the health bill, the financial gains that could be generated for the health care industry are hard to overstate. But the story simply wasn't run.

More curious still was the silence from the majority of the media on the issue of parliamentary links to private health care firms. The *Mirror*'s investigation put the number of Lords with direct interests in NHS privatisation at 40,[22] while the Social Investigations blog suggested that it could be as high as 142.[23] Lord Bell, for instance, is chairman of Chime Communications Group, which includes multiple health care firms. Fleshing out the man beneath the ermine, Social Investigations noted that Bell also 'has a conviction for "wilfully, openly and obscenely" exposing himself "with intent to insult a female" under Section 4 of the 1824 Vagrancy Act'. Then there was Lord Higgins, who according to the *Mirror* held over £50,000 of shares in Lansdowne UK

Equity Fund, a major investor in Circle Holdings. In early 2012 Circle Health, a majority-owned subsidiary, was the first private company to take over an NHS hospital, the Hinchingbrooke.[24] Baroness Bottomley of Nettlestone is a director of BUPA, and Lord Magan is a director of the SISK group of health care companies, to name but a few. The *Mail* and *Telegraph* contained just single mentions of such interests in their respective blog sections rather than in the main 'news' section, while it appears that the *Sun, Independent*, Channel 4 and the BBC never mentioned the issue once; to these outlets, this was a non-story.

An amendment to the health bill was later proposed by Lord Hunt which, according to Channel 4, 'argued that [CCG] members' financial interests should be registered and that anyone flouting the rules should be barred from membership of a Clinical Commissioning Group for up to 10 years'.[25] The assembled Lords, with significant health care links among them, voted down the amendment, 259 votes to 186. Putting strong protections in place against conflicts of interest was mysteriously unpopular. By and large, the British media seemed to agree.

A similar picture emerges when the interests of the honourable Members of the House of Commons are examined. As Sonia Poulton wrote on her blog at the *Daily Mail*: 'At the last count, 31 Lords and 18 MP's have extremely lucrative interests in the health industry – including health providers such as BUPA, pharmaceuticals and consultancies.'[26] With the exception of Poulton and writers for the *Guardian*, no other references appear to have been made by media commentators or reporters about those MPs who had links to the health care industry. No mention was made by the BBC, Channel 4, the *Telegraph, Daily Mail, Independent, Mirror* or *Sun*, as far as research into these outlets' archives has found.

To understand the sort of links in question, Conservative MP Nick de Bois provides a useful illustration. De Bois was on the committee overlooking the health bill's progress and issued a widely reported list of 'red lines' over which he urged the government not to back down, including the clauses opening up the NHS to 'Any Qualified Provider'. De Bois is majority shareholder in Rapier Design Group, which he founded in 1998, and, as the *Guardian* reported: 'Last April, Rapier Design purchased Hampton Medical Conferences to "strengthen the company's position in the medical sector". It is involved in running conferences and other events for private-sector clients, and for NHS hospitals. A number of the company's clients are "partners" of the National Association of Primary Care (NAPC), a lobby group supporting the health secretary's plans.'[27] De Bois's actions came to light when Labour MP Grahame Morris wrote to the Speaker of the House complaining that De Bois's interests had not been disclosed during the passage of the bill. Despite this clear conflict of interest, the *Guardian* was the only media outlet to mention the story.

On the specific issue of Lord Carter of Coles, however, the *Mail* was impressively outspoken.[28] Carter was chairman of the Co-operation and Competition Panel tasked with ensuring fair access to NHS contracts for the private sector. Yet at the same time he was receiving £799,000 a year as chair of McKesson Information Solutions, part of the massive American health care firm McKesson, as well as holding a number of other highly paid positions with health links. As Dr Clare Gerada, chair of the Royal College of General Practitioners, told the *Mail*: 'He cannot have any credibility when he is also heading a company with such huge interests in the very contracts his organisation is meant to police.' Though the *Guardian* picked up the story, the BBC and the rest of the media, once again, ignored it.

The scale of conflicting interests was substantial. Along with MPs' and Lords' financial ties to private health care, there were sizeable donations to the Conservatives from wealthy figures within the industry. There were also clear hazards of GPs and commissioners contracting services from firms they had interests in. As had already been shown, many GPs on the commissioning boards did have financial interests in health care providers. On top of this, it was publicly known that McKinsey had played a direct role in drafting the Health and Social Care Act 2012, despite the likelihood that it would be one of the prime beneficiaries of the newly created health market. The regulator Monitor remains dominated by ex-McKinsey and ex-KPMG staff. Yet, the Health and Social Care Act's labyrinth of vested interests was regularly downplayed in the media and often simply not reported at all. As Channel 4 commented: 'The inter-penetration between the political class, think tanks, lobby groups and private health companies in the UK lies at the heart of some of the criticism of the Coalition's health policies.'[29] At the BBC and much of the press, these links appear to have been consistently ignored.

On some 'vested interests', however, the media were extremely vigilant and explained to the public time and again the murky forces at play. Between the *Mail* and the *Telegraph*, 'vested interests' were raised in news coverage of the bill thirty-four times. In every single case it was not those standing to make substantial profits from the bill that were put under the spotlight but the 'greedy doctors', the BMA, the royal colleges, 'NHS bureaucrats', hospital staff and nurses – in other words, the people running the nation's most valued institution and who were achieving record satisfaction levels and saving countless lives every day. Nor was this completely lost on the public. Comments beneath these articles – including at the *Daily Mail*, hardly a bastion of pro-state sentimentality – made very plain who the real 'vested interests' were in the public's eyes and portrayed an overwhelming sense of anger and grief at what was happening. Many of these comments are still viewable, a document of the failures of the press to answer to the public's interests. As to the combined reporting of 'private', 'corporate', 'commercial' or 'financial interests' in the context of influencing the legislation, the *Mail* and the *Telegraph* return just three results between them – a blog post, an article on Cherie Blair and the *Mail*'s McKinsey scoop.

EXPERTS OR LOBBYISTS?

The firms and individuals pushing for the marketisation of NHS services are perfectly entitled to put their case forward publicly but problems arise when their interests are not made clear to the public and lobbyists are portrayed as disinterested experts. Take 2020health.org, described by the BBC as a 'health think tank': Julia Manning, its chief executive, was twice invited to discuss the NHS on air and a whole article was devoted to covering one of her organisation's reports. At the *Mail*, Manning was given her own blog, where she repeatedly championed Lansley's proposed changes. The blog's byline informed readers that 2020health.org is an 'independent health think tank'. But just how 'independent' was it? Not very, according to SpinWatch, which reported that Tom Sackville, the organisation's chairman and a former Tory minister, 'is CEO of the International Federation of Health Plans, which represents one hundred private health insurance companies in 31 countries'. SpinWatch goes on to disclose that 2020health. org's advisory council 'includes a former director of pharmaceutical giant AstraZeneca, the managing director of bankers NM Rothschild, the past president of the National Pharmaceutical Association, medical director of the Nuffield private hospital group, and CEO of Independent Healthcare Advisory Services, which represents the private healthcare sector'.[30]

Another favourite expert group brought in to give commentary on BBC TV and radio was Reform, an organisation described to the public merely as 'a think tank'. Senior staff at Reform, usually deputy director Nick Seddon, were invited to discuss the health bill with the BBC on five separate occasions. Before joining Reform, Seddon had been head of communications at Circle, the first private health company to take over an NHS hospital, the Hinchingbrooke – yet Seddon's former role was never disclosed by the BBC. Seddon had been replaced at Circle by Christina Lineen, a former aide to Andrew Lansley. To complete the circle, in September 2012 the *Guardian* reported that Jeremy Hunt, Lansley's replacement as Health Secretary, wanted to bring back Lineen as his adviser.[31] The skills needed to promote a private health care company are clearly deemed to be very similar to those required to advise consecutive Coalition health secretaries.

An openDemocracy article noted that: 'Reform's corporate partners represent some of the most powerful companies in the country, including the likes of Citigroup, KPMG, GlaxoSmithKline and Serco.'[32] Many of these partners stand to make substantial profits from the new market created with the Health and Social Care Act 2012. Through Seddon's and other Reform staff's appearances, the BBC may have facilitated private sector lobbying on a publicly funded platform without making relevant interests known. Channel 4, in contrast, presented Reform with full disclosure as to the organisation's mission and key staff links with private health care interests.

Reform ran a very successful press operation in its efforts to lobby for the bill. The *Telegraph* allowed senior Reform staff to write regularly for the paper: director Andrew Haldenby appears to have written at least six articles while the bill was going through Parliament,[33] and Nick Seddon a further two. The readers of these articles were informed that Reform is an 'independent think tank', though, as the word 'independent' is usually understood by the general public, its use here may have been somewhat misleading. It is worth noting a leaked document from David Worskett, director of NHS Partners Network – an alliance of private health firms – passed to Social Investigations, dated 20 May 2011. It contained the following boast from Worskett: 'And the whole sequence of *Telegraph* articles and editorials on the importance of the Government not going soft on public service reform, including some strong pieces on health, is something I have been orchestrating and working with Reform to bring about.'[34] While Max Pemberton's excellent 'Life on the NHS frontline' blog at the *Telegraph* did provide readers with a countering, authoritative voice on the issues, publishing health care lobbyists without making their connections clear seems misjudged, particularly when the pieces were published in the heart of the 'listening' pause – the moment when influences of this sort had the most chance to affect the legislation's future. Seddon's two articles, for instance, appeared on 16 May ('David Cameron is getting it wrong on NHS reform', which was subtitled 'The NHS is crying out for greater choice' and referenced six Reform studies on 'successful private sector involvement'[35]) and 18 May ('Why the NHS needs a regulator'[36] – a piece championing the idea that Monitor needed to be focused on competition as much as patient health).

At the BBC opportunities were frequently missed to provide expert opposition to the bill on a consistent basis. The RCGP's Clare Gerada was largely the exception to the rule. Many of the most well-known and authoritative critics of the bill – the likes of professors Allyson Pollock or Colin Leys, doctors Jacky Davis and Wendy Savage from Keep Our NHS Public (some of whom are contributors to this volume) – never appeared on the BBC to discuss the plans. Davis recalls being invited to appear on the BBC a number of times but the item was cancelled on every occasion. 'Balance' is supposedly one of the BBC's primary objectives yet appearing on the *Today* programme of 1 February 2012 to discuss the bill, for instance, were Shirley Williams (who voted in favour of the bill, however reluctantly), Nick Seddon of 'independent' Reform (pro-bill), Steve Field (pro-bill) and Chris Ham (pro-bill). It's difficult to see how that is not a breach of BBC guidelines and a disservice to the public. One of the fundamental duties of an open media is to ensure that coverage is not skewed towards those with the deepest pockets. And on that issue the media often performed poorly.

Further criticism of the BBC stems from its curious lack of NHS coverage during the climactic final month before the bill was passed in the House of Lords on 19 March. One such complaint came from blogger and Oxford Professor of Developmental Neuropsychology Dorothy Bishop, who wrote to the BBC to ask why it had failed to cover a number of NHS stories in March, including an anti-bill petition that had been brought to the House by Lord Owen, carrying 486,000 signatures of support.[37] In reply, the BBC confirmed that the bill had been mentioned on the *Today* programme in March prior to the bill's passing, though just once. Bishop replied: 'So, if I have understood this right, during March, the *Today* programme covered the story once, in an early two-minute slot, before the bill was passed. Other items that morning included four minutes on a French theme park based on Napoleon, six minutes on international bagpipe day and eight minutes on Jubilee celebrations.'[38]

Other BBC omissions include Andrew Lansley being heckled by angry medical staff at a hospital in Hampstead, as reported by both the *Mail* and Sky News. On 17 March a peaceful anti-bill march took place in central London. Those out protesting for their national health service found themselves kettled by riot police despite being one of the most harmless-looking crowds you're ever likely to see. The protest and the shameful police response were completely ignored by the media, except for a brief mention on a *Guardian* blog. On social media numerous examples have been reported of protests and actions opposing the bill that were entirely absent from national coverage.

Then, on 19 March, the day of the final vote on the bill, the BBC ran not a single article on the event, despite this being one of the most bitterly opposed pieces of legislation in recent history – it was as if the vote was not taking place. The next day, with the bill passed, they ran a full seven articles on the story. Three days after the bill passed, Radio 4 broadcast *The Report*: 'Simon Cox asks: why is NHS reform mired in controversy?' Why this was not broadcast before the Lords vote is a mystery.

'GP COMMISSIONING'

Explaining what the bill would mean for the NHS and for the public's health was not easy. But, as a number of organisations proved, it was far from an impossible task. Time and again, however, the BBC summarised the bill in almost identical fashion: 'the bill will give control of most of the NHS budget to GPs and there will be a greater role for the private and voluntary sectors'. On the day the bill was passed, the bulletin scrolling across the *BBC News* screen stated: 'Bill which gives power to GPs passes'.

Similar formulations were evident in much of the media, not only the BBC, and the failure to explain the basics of the bill and why it was opposed led to some bewildering articles. For instance, the following from *Sky News*, which included the assessment under the headline, 'Lansley: My stroke influenced NHS reforms':

> Mr Lansley wants to give GPs a much bigger say in the
> provision of services but has been forced to reconsider
> his plans after a backlash from health workers and the
> public. At a Royal College of Nursing annual meeting
> a week ago, 92% of delegates supported a vote of no
> confidence in him.[39]

The media almost daily found themselves explaining a health bill
that 'aimed to give power to GPs and frontline staff' yet was
bitterly opposed by those very GPs and frontline health staff,
not to mention the unions, public health academics and nearly
all of the royal colleges. Something wasn't quite adding up. The
government faced similar problems: one minute Lansley was
'empowering GPs' to take control and the next dismissing their
opposition on the basis of their 'vested interests'. With a £60
billion to £80 billion budget to play with, and endless empowerment on the way, the readers of the nation's newspapers may
have been confused to learn that the RCGP overwhelmingly
rejected the bill.[40]

At the root of the media's problem was a failure to explain the
scope of the bill or the reasons *why* it was so vehemently opposed.
Turning the NHS into a full-blooded, competitive market open
to 'Any Qualified Provider' and allowing up to 49 per cent of
NHS hospitals to be used for private patients, for instance, were
frequently described in reports as simply 'an increased role for the
private sector'. Criticisms would be noted as 'fears of creeping
privatisation', without properly explaining why such fears existed
or how likely they were to materialise.

The idea that opposition to the bill was too complex or fragmented to summarise effectively was simply untrue. Here is an
adapted Keep Our NHS Public (KONP) briefing, for instance:

Opponents claim the bill has no electoral mandate and it will end the comprehensive system free to all patients when they need it. They say private companies, the voluntary sector and NHS hospitals will compete in a 'regulated' market with no requirement to provide healthcare for all. GPs will commission care from 'any qualified provider' with accountants, lawyers, and multinational firms heavily involved. The bill will also allow Foundation Trust hospitals to earn up to half their income from treating private patients.

Or as Channel 4 explained:

[Critics] have also raised questions as to the motives which underpin what appears to be the partial privatisation of a major public institution. And this has in turn shone the spotlight on Andrew Lansley himself, his background and his connections. The inter-penetration between the political class, think tanks, lobby groups and private health companies in the UK lies at the heart of some of the criticism of the Coalition's health policies.[41]

In addition, the Health and Social Care Act 2012 formally removed the Secretary of State's 'duty to provide comprehensive healthcare' – the legal foundation of the NHS since 1948 – leaving only the duty to 'promote'. This aspect of the bill appears to have received only one or two mentions in most of the media, and none at all in some papers. For the BBC and other media to routinely describe the bill as 'giving power to GPs and allowing a greater role for the private sector' amounts to little more than regurgitating government press releases.

POWER PLAYERS

What the public may find most surprising in the media coverage of the health bill is the pattern of shortcomings, the lack of interest in vital parts of the story across the spectrum, from the right-wing *Daily Mail* and *Telegraph* to the supposedly 'left-of-centre' BBC and *Independent*. There were a few exceptions: the *Guardian* and Channel 4 consistently showed the candour and commitment that an issue as important as the future of the NHS deserves. The wider coverage, however, often failed in the press's duty to inform and educate.

Considering that the *Sun* is read by millions of people per day – the largest circulation in the UK, and the tenth largest in the world – the newspaper's measly output on the proposed changes to the NHS is quite shocking. Of the twenty-four stories on the health bill that were tracked for press coverage for this chapter's analysis, the *Sun* covered a total of zero. But, then again, as News International's Rebekah Brooks famously assured David Cameron, they were 'all in it together'.

Campaigners may not expect more from the *Sun* but they certainly do from the BBC, given its status as an impartial public service broadcaster whose news-gathering is supported directly by licence-fee payers. The BBC accounts for 70 per cent of news consumption on television.[42] Further, the BBC accounts for 40 per cent of online news read by the public, three times that of its closest competitor, the *Mail*. Quite simply, the BBC dominates UK news. The weight given to the BBC here is not purely down to its dominance, however, but also because, along with the NHS, the BBC remains one of our great public institutions, an entity that is supposedly above commercial pressures. Many of the stories ignored by the BBC were covered by the for-profit, right-wing press, as well as the *Guardian* and Channel 4, so the concern is not that the organisation failed to 'campaign' for the NHS, but that it failed to report facts that other outlets found newsworthy.

The BBC's archive of TV and radio coverage is neither available for the public to research nor technically practical to research, but there are a number of reasons for confidence that their online content is highly indicative of their broader output. First, BBC Online is a fully integrated part of the main newsroom rather than a separate operation. Consequently, TV and radio coverage that can be examined is largely indistinguishable from the related online content, as demonstrated in the examples given above. During the debate of Lansley's bill, BBC TV and radio were both subject to multiple complaints, the figures for which the BBC has declined to release.

Broadsheet coverage was flawed in similar ways. The *Independent*, *Daily Mail* and *Telegraph*, for instance, all published some excellent pieces of journalism about the White Paper and the health bill, and it would be misleading to suggest they gave the government an easy ride. They didn't. But there were some common problems. All three papers supported the bill in their editorials and that editorial support was paired with a lack of reporting in a number of relevant areas.[43] Stories that brought the legitimacy and propriety of the bill into question were often overlooked, particularly at the *Independent*. Stories were often presented in isolation, or linked to inadequate summaries of the bill and the opposition to its proposed reforms. Those incidents that were covered tended to be just as quickly forgotten and rarely did they appear in the summaries; they were not part of the *ongoing narrative* presented to readers. Too often, critical details were submerged by media preference for Westminster chit-chat about who said what; but what those in power are *saying* is not always the same thing as what those in power are *doing*. It's often quite the opposite. The bill was typically presented in a very charitable light and lobbyists and government spokespeople appeared to have enjoyed considerable access to both the BBC and broadsheets, often without proper disclosure.

Donations, lobbying, conflicts of interest, close links between Westminster, think tanks and the private sector, the role of the private sector in pushing for the bill and having a role in drafting elements of it – omitting these elements from the media coverage concealed something quite fundamental, namely that the Health and Social Care Act was primarily motivated by commercial interests. This wildly unpopular, brazen and dishonest raid on the nation's most valued institution was a gross breach of the democratic contract. Something was driving it forward, through opposition, pause and emergency motions – and that something was neither the public nor the medical professions.

Notwithstanding the media reticence on key issues, a substantial proportion of the public did have a grasp of the broader implications of Lansley's plans and, when asked, they rejected the framing adopted by the Coalition Government and mirrored in the media. Public opposition to the bill remained consistently high: protests, candle-lit vigils, marathons and local campaigns took place all over the country, though virtually none of this activity was reported on the BBC or in the press. Even at the right-wing *Mail*, the most popular readers' comments that appeared beneath the articles expressed outrage at the bill. Over and over, these comments conveyed dismay at what readers saw as privatisation of a public service at the hands of private interests.

One explanation for this divergence of public and media views is that the extent to which the public rely on the national media to form their views is overstated, a position supported by much academic research on the issue. By 2009 – that is, before the News International phone-hacking scandal broke – public trust in journalists had fallen to just 19 per cent, only marginally higher than the figure for politicians, who came in at 17 per cent.[44]

It should also be remembered that the public have now had thirty years' experience of the privatisation of state assets and services, as well as the rhetoric that accompanies such moves, and they are increasingly cynical about the purported aims and efficacy of such 'reforms'. Margaret Thatcher spent millions of pounds marketing her privatisations to the public, yet polling revealed that support for this policy never rose above 50 per cent.[45] In the wake of the Iraq War, the expenses revelations, the financial crash and the phone-hacking scandal, public trust in the political class as a whole, including in the national media, is extremely low.

As many in both the government and the media could agree, the NHS reforms were also 'badly communicated'. The public may have disliked the sound of them, but they 'didn't understand them'. In some respects, the reforms were explained *too openly* and the public understood them all too well. Loose talk from health care executives and ministers, and revelations from old policy papers, were pounced upon and hauled into the public square. Andrew Lansley, lacking the 'communication skills' of PR men like Tony Blair or David Cameron, never really managed to gain control of the discourse. The reforms were simply too vast, they affected too many workers and professions, too many organisations, and the NHS is one of the few services used by nearly everyone.

Control of information is also weakening. Sources such as Social Investigations and SpinWatch published major investigations while campaigners such as Keep Our NHS Public increasingly utilised social media to distribute briefings and materials without having to navigate the traditional media gatekeepers. Though the Health and Social Care Act may have passed, it was and still is bitterly opposed.

The overall media coverage of the health bill brings to mind a quote from BBC radio correspondent Nicholas Jones, on the BBC's coverage of the miners' strike: 'stories that gave prominence to the position of the National Union of Miners could simply be omitted, shortened, or submerged into another report'.[46] The apparent unwillingness of the media to challenge the impropriety surrounding the bill remains disturbing, if not surprising. Any lingering doubts as to the closeness of many parts of the media to government were finally swept away with the Murdoch scandal and the Leveson inquiry that followed. In outlook, too, both the commercial media and Westminster share a largely consistent pro-market agenda. The end result is that while Parliament's 'bad apples' may be ruthlessly hounded, questioning the integrity of our wider political system *itself*, and particularly its co-option by market interests, is still regarded to be 'ungentlemanly' and somehow crass. The health bill, a near perfect vision of Westminster's appropriation by high commerce, only made the disparity between reality and reporting all the more stark.

7

FROM CRADLE TO GRAVE

Allyson M. Pollock and David Price

People will die because of the Government's decision to
focus on competition rather than quality in health care.

Richard Horton, editor of *The Lancet*

At 2.36p.m. on the afternoon of Tuesday, 27 March 2012, immediately after prayers from the Lord Bishop of Ripon and Leeds,
the Health and Social Care Bill repealing the legal foundations
of the NHS in England was given royal assent and became law.
It was a dry and formal end to a tumultuous parliamentary passage, for as we have seen in the preceding chapters, the bill had
not reached the statute book without a struggle. Campaigning
groups and NHS staff and professional organisations had fought
for nearly all of the previous two years against what is one of the
most regressive pieces of legislation in the UK over the last sixty
years. Promoted using the rhetoric of 'patient choice', in reality
the bill challenged tax-funded health care and public provision

by introducing structures borrowed from an American insurance industry notorious for its high cost and inequalities.

Rarely can a reform have traded under colours as false as this. That the bill became law in the end is testimony not to our robust democratic processes, but to the autocratic power of government. The Coalition came to office in May 2010 on a manifesto promising no further 'top-down' reform of the NHS, and then promptly did the opposite. The Labour Party's own market-reform record contained many elements such as the privatisation of clinical care that were now being implemented with renewed vigour by the Coalition. This stifled the presumed partisan opposition.

The bill passed into law without an electoral mandate, because no major political party or parliamentary institution in England was willing or able to defend the NHS. It was a constitutional outrage. Its passing marked the end of a national health service in England that for nearly sixty-five years has served as one of the most successful models of health care in the world – widely praised and much copied.

The NHS had risen to be an international model because it provided what no other country in the world has been able to achieve at the same cost: universal health care in the form of equal access to comprehensive care irrespective of personal income. For most of its existence the NHS was based on the principle that the poor, the chronically sick and the frail elderly would receive the best available care *only if* the rich received the same service. Since the 1970s and throughout the 1980s and '90s we have witnessed a dismantling of publicly funded long-term care, including nursing care for the elderly; huge inequalities have accompanied these brutalities. The Health and Social Care Act 2012 is a prelude to the adoption of the same stratagems for hospital and primary care, in the most succinct terms, because it repeals the law ensuring that everyone, rich or poor, wherever they live, receives the same health care.

How can we make such bold statements? The duty of the Secretary of State has been, until this point, to secure or provide comprehensive health services – the government responsibility for universal health care rests with this office. But, with the passing of the health bill, that duty has been abolished. This is why, we argue, the reinstatement of that duty must be the cornerstone of any plan to undo the catastrophic policy adopted by the Coalition Government and save the NHS.

FAIR SHARES FOR ALL

When the NHS was ushered into existence on 5 July 1948, it provided the entire population of the UK with health care free at the point of delivery. Its aim was to treat all alike on the basis of need, not the ability to pay. Charity, market-based provision and National Insurance schemes had failed to deliver the universal health care that the nation required. In the 1930s only 43 per cent of the population were covered by the National Insurance scheme: these lucky minority were mainly men and they only qualified to receive general practitioner services. More than twenty-one million people, mainly women and children, were not covered at all, and the sick carried the burden of paying for their care.

It was not until the Second World War, when Churchill's government created the emergency bed and medical services, which brought all hospitals under government control, that the population got a taste of universal health care. So the NHS was created out of a national consensus to ensure that every citizen was guaranteed health care. For the first time, the population as a whole would enjoy 'freedom from fear' – and, above all, freedom from the costs of ill health.

The NHS was only one of the pillars of the new, postwar welfare state. As Sir William Beveridge scathingly noted, 'want is a needless scandal due to not taking the trouble to prevent it – it is well within the economic resources of the country to prevent it'. During the war years he had been asked by the government to work on a plan for eradicating what he termed the five 'giants': ignorance, idleness, want, disease and squalor. His report, entitled *The Plan for Social Security and Allied Social Services*,[1] was published in 1944 and sold out within twenty-four hours. It bequeathed to a nation, worn out from war, a huge programme of reform, which would bring public services to the forefront of redistribution, equity and a more just society. Thus, the reform programme and the NHS became a model for public services across much of the Western world.

The architects of the NHS recognised that equity in health care could only be achieved by sharing the risks and costs of care across the whole of society, from rich to poor and from healthy to sick. It is well established that poverty and ill health are closely associated. The poor have higher rates of sickness and illness than the wealthy. Risk sharing means that those with the highest needs must not be penalised for being both sick and poor. It was for this reason that the architects of the NHS embedded solidarity and collective provision into the structures for the funding and delivery of care.[2]

Whilst a commitment to central taxation was seen as the most progressive and efficient way of pooling the costs of health care, it was also recognised that services must be integrated so that patients could not be denied care or passed from one service to another to save money or avoid high-cost individuals. The higher costs of delivering services to rural communities must be shared with urban communities, because access to services and costs of supplying services is greater in more remote areas. Expensive treatments or rare conditions, such as bone marrow transplants and blood transfusion services, require service integration and risk sharing so that the less expensive parts of the service or investigations subsidise the more expensive. When a patient is admitted for a routine operation and requires ventilation and intensive care, the cost of this treatment would be spread across the whole system.

Integration was enshrined in the system. Public administration ruled out the division of services into separate 'profit' opportunities, which would inevitably prevent cross-subsidisation. It also ruled out the inefficiencies associated with billing, invoicing and marketing. Furthermore, administration was based on geographical units, originally known as regional and district health boards, which covered all citizens resident within them and to which resources were channelled on the basis of measurements of the whole population's health care needs. No one was to be excluded.

A DUTY TO PROVIDE

Underpinning these arrangements was the Secretary of State's core duty to provide or secure a comprehensive health service – the duty repealed by the first clause of the Health and Social Care Act 2012. This repeal was the fulcrum of the free-market agenda, since this long-standing duty compelled the minister to allocate resources according to need instead of leaving allocation to market forces and unaccountable organisations.

The duty had originated in 1946, along with the beginning of the government's responsibility for provision to the whole population of all medical, dental and nursing care. Sections 1 and 3 of the National Health Service Act 1946 required the Minister of Health to promote free of charge 'the establishment in England and Wales of a comprehensive health service for the prevention, diagnosis and treatment of illness' and to do so by providing 'to such extent as he considers necessary to meet all reasonable requirements … (a) hospital accommodation; (b) medical, nursing and other services required at or for the purposes of hospitals; (c) the services of specialists, whether at a hospital, a health centre ... or a clinic or, if necessary on medical grounds, at the home of the patient.'[3]

These essential legal principles were to remain unchanged for more than sixty years and, following the introduction of equivalent legislation in Scotland, they ensured equitable and comprehensive health care throughout the UK. The principles were essential because a minister may only be held to account legally for services that he or she is responsible for by law. Their repeal was a hugely controversial moment in the history of the NHS. No previous reform, and there have been many, had been designed to abolish this national principle, although many inroads had been made into the structures necessary to deliver it.

The determination of the government to push the legal change through in the face of a barrage of criticism served only to underline the strategic nature of the measure: that the proposed market system was inconsistent with the founding duty of the NHS. Quite simply, markets do not and cannot deliver equitable, comprehensive health care; that is not what they are for. The government, given a duty to provide comprehensive health care to the whole population, was required to design an administrative system that would allow it to discharge that responsibility. Such a system would be inclusive, covering everyone. If the duty were to be the promotion of a market, the structures that would follow would be those consistent with the commercial strategies of market actors, namely the freedom to select services and patients on commercial grounds. If markets were to be introduced, the universal provision duty had to go.

Legal functions are therefore key to health system structures, which is why the Coalition Government, throughout the long parliamentary debates, stuck fast to its repeal of the duty to provide. The classification of health systems according to their method of financing has tended to obscure this fundamental fact. Traditionally, health systems have been distinguished according to how they raise money.

Since 1948 most funding for health care in the UK has been raised through general taxes. Individuals and businesses are not mandated to contribute to the costs of health care, except as part of their general duty to pay taxes. Instead, the government is mandated to provide universal health care free at the point of delivery.

Financing methods reflect the laws defining government responsibilities and the structures that governments put in place to discharge them. Tax-financed systems are associated with directly managed health care facilities rather than commercial contracting methods of control. Most NHS-type systems around the world are based on a mandate similar to the UK's, and on administrative structures designed to allocate health care resources according to need. The NHS approach has served as an international model because it has proved to be the most efficient and surest route to universal access yet discovered.

Distinctive administrative functions flow from the Secretary of State's duty to provide health care to all, along with the government's assumption of responsibility for the costs of comprehensive health care to the entire population. As a result, the focus shifts to health service planning, needs assessment and resource allocation across geographic populations in order that no one slips through the net or goes without care, an approach pioneered in the NHS. The NHS system has thus encouraged extensive data collection and analysis on population health, health inequalities and access to health care by social class and ethnicity.

The approach is entirely different in market systems. Here, financial risks are allocated across different parts of the system through market contracting, and there is no duty to provide services on a comprehensive basis or to collect data on a geographic basis. Instead, administrative functions in market systems focus on risk pricing and segmentation across providers, members or enrollees. It was such a system that the Health and Social Care Act was intended to bring in, primarily through the attack on 'systemic' NHS 'red tape'.

THE ATTACK ON 'RED TAPE'

From 1948 to 2012 the NHS was the vehicle whereby the government was made responsible by Parliament for providing equitable health care. However, a succession of statutory changes increasingly undermined each government's capacity to carry out this function efficiently, especially so far as hospitals were concerned. Market-orientated reforms began in 1990 with the introduction of a purchaser–provider split and the new approach of 'commissioning' (sometimes known as the 'internal' market, as mentioned earlier in this book). Commissioning meant that hospitals were expected to compete with one another for NHS funds under a system where instead of receiving block grants 'money followed patients'. Eventually, in 2000, the hospitals were paid on the basis of the work and patients they could attract from other hospitals – the more work they got, the more money they received. Then, in 2003, NHS hospitals which had already been established in 1990 as stand-alone corporate bodies with their own balance sheets were to be transformed into 'foundation trusts'. Foundation trusts were put beyond ministerial control so as to give market forces more influence over hospital policy and they were given new freedoms to generate income from private patients and run businesses jointly with commercial companies.[4]

Opportunities for contracting-out clinical care gradually increased in other parts of the health system. In 2004 the new GP contract gave primary care trusts (PCTs) and GPs permission to contract out clinical services through commercial providers, and in 2005 authorities began to buy non-emergency surgery from newly established independent treatment centres, many of which were commercially owned and run. By 2008 the Department of Health began to experiment with a policy of full competition on the provider side.

Whereas most of the changes prior to Andrew Lansley's reforms in 2012 involved reducing government control over the various components of the health system and creating measures to divert NHS funding to the corporate sector, the new health act went for the fundamental control mechanism, namely the contiguous area-based system of public administration. That system had served for nearly sixty-five years as a means for keeping expenditures under control whilst seeking to ensure resources were efficiently distributed according to need and the duty to provide comprehensive cover throughout England.

Within weeks of the 2010 general election, the Coalition Government laid out its plans to 'liberate' the NHS. The 'natural condition of organisations', it proclaimed, 'ought to be freedom rather than being shackled'.[5] A fact sheet was published to hammer home the message:

> We're moving away from top-down organisation and control. We're removing targets that tie up NHS staff in red tape and we're getting politicians out of decision-making. We're removing whole tiers of management that sit above doctors and nurses and instead giving them the power to decide what's best for their patients. We're giving patients more choice and control over their care, rather than managers telling them what they get. Our changes are about simplifying and modernising the NHS; not top-down change.[6]

The inclusion of patient choice in the message had become the standard way of promoting market over government control.

Removal of these administrative tiers depended on abolition of the Secretary of State's duty to provide, because, so long as the duty remained in place, the government would have to ensure continuation of a broadly similar administrative system and cover for all. The act therefore took market reform further than previous governments by abolishing the main administrative tier through which universality had been assured. The change was achieved by absolving the government from responsibility for the full financial risk of health care and by devolving it on to CCGs, local authorities, providers, the public and, ultimately, patients. An administrative system dedicated purely to the government bearing the risk of universal access and equity was no longer required in law.

The reform also involved abolition of PCTs, the purpose of which had been to ensure that all people throughout the country were covered and that health services were organised on a geographical basis. PCTs were the outward and visible sign of the government's duty to ensure all citizens received the same care. Their abolition was central to the creation of a new system in which the government ceased to underwrite the principle of equal care for equal need. CCGs are not the same as PCTs; their structures are drawn from insurance funds, where entitlement is not automatic as it has been for all residents throughout England, but depends upon proof of membership. Initially members will be drawn from GP practice lists, which in turn have more freedom to enrol and disenrol patients based on risk..

The whole reform package was sold as a means of doing essentially the same as before but using competition or patient choice, rather than administrative controls, to do it more efficiently. Following economic theory, the Coalition Government argued that, in an ideal world, external or market pressure was necessary to prevent providers pursuing their own interests, hospitals admitting more patients than necessary and doctors prescribing or referring patients to hospital without proper regard for costs. The reality and the evidence, however, contradict the theory.

DUTY, FULLY REPEALED

The Coalition Government's approach to the legislative process and their policy rationale were less than candid. In fact, as we have seen in some detail throughout this book, they bordered on flagrant misrepresentation. But, for a start, the enormity of the change was only apparent to those capable of understanding draft legislation. The health bill began: '(1) Section 1 of the National Health Service Act 2006 [Secretary of State's duty to promote health service] is amended as follows. (2) For subsection (2) sub-stitute –'. Subsection 2 of the 2006 Act read: '(2) The Secretary of State must for that purpose provide or secure the provision of services in accordance with this Act.'[7]

Contrast this with the duty to provide comprehensive health services throughout England and Wales in the 1946 act that cre-ated the NHS. It read: '(1) It shall be the duty of the Minister of Health ... to promote the establishment in England and Wales of a comprehensive health service ... and for that purpose to provide or secure the effective provision of services in accordance with the following provisions of this Act.' By 2006, the wording, though slightly weakened and modified, remained broadly the same: '(1) The Secretary of State must continue the promotion in England of a comprehensive health service ... (2) The Secretary of State must for that purpose provide or secure the provision of services in accordance with this Act.' In both cases, the phrase 'in accordance with this act' was a reference to a comprehensive health service.

At the start, the enormity of the change was only apparent to those capable of understanding draft legislation. In contrast to the stark and honest simplicity of the 1946 legislation and the leaflet that went to every household to explain it, Lansley's bill and its roll out seemed deliberately designed to conceal its true purpose.

Lansley's bill was a complicated and almost unintelligible read, certainly for those not trained in legal analysis, but what matters was that its revisions accomplished the abolition of the original duty of the Secretary of State that had been included in legislation since the inception of the NHS. Scarcely can such a fundamental change of duty have been so little advertised or explained – but then, this was not a measure the government wanted to trumpet. And the Coalition's repeated denials that any change of substance would come if the bill were enacted made the task of interpretation harder still. When the bill reached the House of Lords, its champion there, Earl Howe, would tell another peer that the legislation was 'vital' but 'in practice … will change little'.[8]

However, thanks to the work of barrister Peter Roderick, who worked with us and other colleagues at Queen Mary, University of London, to dissect the meaning of the health bill, the government's true intentions were exposed – to those who were willing to see them. During the final six months during which the bill was discussed and passed through the Lords, we at Queen Mary published fifteen detailed legal and public health briefings and several academic articles on its changes and their implications, laying bare the government's intentions. The government attacked us and rejected our analysis but was unable to say *why* they insisted that we were wrong.

Indeed, as has been outlined elsewhere in this book, the government could not silence a number of important critics – most especially Dr Clare Gerada, the chair of the powerful Royal College of General Practitioners (RCGP), which represents the majority of GPs, the very doctors who, according to the government, would be at the helm of CCGs and thus responsible for the allocation of NHS funds. Gerada warned of the perils that lay ahead. Nor could the government quell the growing public and political storm.

Various alterations were made to the duty of provision as the bill wound its way through committees of the House of Commons and House of Lords in an attempt to placate these critics. But the amendments were mainly cosmetic and offered no real concessions. Abolition of the duty to provide turned out to be a government red line, a measure it simply refused to give up. By 3 February 2012, 239 amendments had been tabled to the Health and Social Care Bill to be moved on report. Of these, 165 (mainly government) amendments were tabled on 1 February 2012. By the time the Lords voted through the bill, clause 1 provided that, for the purpose of promoting a comprehensive health service, the Secretary of State 'must exercise the functions conferred by this Act so as to secure that services are provided in accordance with this Act'. As we have seen, this was a pale reminder of the original wording; it echoed the phrases without clearly maintaining a free-standing duty. The bill did not lay down a duty on the Secretary of State to secure provision of health services, only a duty to exercise other functions to secure provision. So, if the other functions conferred by the act did not impose a duty on the Secretary of State to provide or secure provision, then he or she would have no duty to provide or to secure provision. Since another clause in the bill removed the Secretary of State's duty to provide key listed services as enshrined in the National Health Service Act 2006, the legal duty to provide services effectively disappeared.

The legal link between the minister and health care provision was thus broken and replaced by a series of limited, discretionary powers. As ministers cannot be responsible to Parliament for the exercise of functions that are not theirs, in future, MPs wanting to make recommendations to governments to improve services to patients would only have a miscellany of distant levers to pull. At best, there was to be a line of accountability between Parliament and the public newly set up by the bill (and to which many of the former duties of the Secretary of State were to be transferred). But as a House of Lords Committee wrote in its report on the bill:

> [T]here is a constitutionally significant difference between ministerial responsibility to Parliament and the accountability of a public body (such as the NHS Commissioning Board) to a minister. In constitutional terms the latter can never be a substitute for the former because, in the latter case, Parliament is not involved. As the Minister correctly stated in his opening speech in the second reading debate, 'We in Parliament can only turn to the Secretary of State'. Parliament cannot call or hold the Chair of the Commissioning Board, for example, to constitutional account. A select committee can of course call him as a witness, but giving evidence as a witness to a committee and being liable to be held to account by Parliament are not the same thing.[9]

Should the provisions of the act remain intact, Parliament will not be able in future to hold the Secretary of State to account for failures in the provision of health services in the way it has until now, because there would be no legal duty to do so. Instead, MPs, Lords and select committees will have to rely on a watered-down duty to promote a comprehensive health service, an emergency power of intervention and several discretionary powers. In future, without a stand-alone duty to secure provision, select committees wanting to make recommendations to governments to improve services to patients will only be able to bring indirect pressures to bear.

The effect is to transform the NHS from a nationally mandated public service required of the government into a service based on commercial contracting, underpinned by ministerial and local discretion and exacerbated by a lack of accountability to Parliament of both commissioners and providers. Abolition of the duty of the Secretary of State to provide or secure provision of health services was the seminal change that allowed this transformation to be wrought.

Repeal was not a flaw that could be remedied in isolation but a direct consequence of the policy to abandon a system of health care delivered by public bodies generally acting under statutory duties. The bill introduced a more discretionary and more market-based system in which the minister is at a remove from the services delivered to patients. It was, as Lord Owen pointed out, an 'abdication bill'. This simple difference was lost in a debate that descended into farce, with the government deliberately conflating the abolition of its duties and powers with eliminating political micro-management of health care. That was always a travesty, but it served to distract attention from the knock-on effects of deregulation.

THE ABOLITION OF THE NHS[10]

Repeal of the Secretary of State's duty to secure or provide health services and its replacement by the weaker duty to 'act with a view to securing' comprehensive services also facilitated abolition of the Health Secretary's general powers of direction over NHS bodies and providers. Instead of controlling the health service, the minister's role will in future be focused on public health functions, which become the responsibility of local authorities. Significant consequences follow on from that change, as listed below.

First, new commissioning groups may determine who gets publicly financed care. For example, the act repealed the Health Secretary's duty to 'provide [certain health services] throughout England, to such extent as he considers necessary to meet all reasonable requirements'. Instead, the new clinical commissioning groups (CCGs), responsible for patients from general practices and not areas, will 'arrange for' the services necessary 'to meet all reasonable requirements' and determine which services are 'appropriate as parts of the health service'. A commissioning group does not have a duty to provide a comprehensive range of services but only 'such services or facilities as it considers appropriate'. Nor must it arrange comprehensive services for all persons living in its area.

CCGs will be responsible to the new NHS Commissioning Board (NHSCB), or NHS England as it was renamed in April 2013. NHS England will not have a power of general direction over those health services for which consortiums contract, or over patients' entitlements. Providers of health services will be subject to the 'independent' regulator Monitor. But, like the CCGs, Monitor will not have a duty to ensure provision for all residents or to ensure equity of access and coverage. Monitor's general duty is only to 'protect and promote the interests of people who use health care services'. The commissioning group's duty to arrange for health service provision applies to their enrolled population, that is, the patients on the lists of the general practices that make up the group, not all residents living within a defined geographical area. Full implementation of the 'patient choice' agenda, the banner under which reform was promoted, will mean that general practices, and therefore CCGs, will be able to accept patients regardless of where they live. Practices and commissioning groups will therefore be able to compete (and advertise) for patients from across the whole country, just as private health care corporations and health insurers do now. They will, of course, also be able to reject costly patients.

Second, local authorities will become providers of last resort. Because the Secretary of State will no longer be able to ensure comprehensive, universal cover to all residents in geographically defined areas, the legislators have drafted a safety net whereby local authorities can be required to undertake NHS functions. Under the Health and Social Care Act 2012, the Health Secretary can require councils to provide 'services or facilities for the prevention, diagnosis or treatment of illness'. Local authorities alone have a duty to provide for geographical populations. Health care services that CCGs and market providers deem will threaten their financial viability can therefore be transferred out of the NHS in much the same way as long-term care and continuing care responsibilities were transferred out in 1990. Patients who cannot get access to general practices or the services of CCGs may have to default to local authorities, which would become the provider of last resort. The core functions of the Health Secretary will shift to the chargeable local authority sector.[11]

Third, loss of equity of access will result. The Secretary of State does not have a duty to promote equity of access apart from a vague duty to 'have regard to the need to reduce inequalities between the people of England with respect to the benefits that they can obtain from the health service'. Bizarrely, NHS England will not have a general power of direction over consortiums or be under a duty to ensure equal access for equal need to health services. A vague equity duty also applies to CCGs in the form of a requirement to 'have regard to the need to reduce inequalities between patients'. Equality of access is not a required outcome of CCGs' duty to secure 'continuous improvement' from the provision of services; nor is it part of annual 'commissioning plans' that groups will be required to prepare. These will cover only continuous improvement – and the financial duty to break even.

Fourth, the duty to provide services free of charge will no longer exist. There are new mechanisms to introduce charges and privately funded health care. The Secretary of State's duty to provide free services that are 'part of the health service in England', except where charges are expressly allowed, is undermined because the power under the Health and Medicines Act 1988 to impose charges is transferred from the Secretary of State to commissioning groups – the new CCGs. So CCGs will determine which services are part of the health service and which are chargeable, and they have been given a general power to charge. And as we have seen, the cap on foundation trusts' generation of income from private care is also raised, allowing them to earn almost half their income from non-NHS patients.

Fifth, this leads to the abolition of direct control over NHS provision. The new CCGs are being established as budget holders and will determine which primary and secondary services they contract, from whom and at what cost. Patients may therefore be exposed to a plurality of primary and secondary care contractors for different services. All general practices will be required to join a CCG. Various bodies can apply to become a commissioning group, including foundation trusts and for-profit organisations that run general practices.

Increasingly, general practice and commissioning functions will be operated and managed by for-profit companies, twenty-three of which – including well-established outfits Virgin Care, Care UK and ChilversMcCrae Healthcare – already run 227 general practices. Professional autonomy will be eroded if, for example, referral management centres run by corporate providers are used to ensure referral and prescribing practices conform to corporate budgets and the needs of shareholders. These centres were already rejecting one in eight general practitioner referrals before the full force of the new health law has been felt, and they seem to be operating along the lines of American-style 'prior authorisation' arrangements, whereby doctors are required to obtain approval from a higher authority (usually a private health insurance provider) before making a referral for treatment or investigation. Some of the centres, such as UnitedHealth Group UK's recently established 'referral facilitation service' based in Hounslow, are run by subsidiaries of US health care multinationals.

Sixth, NHS trusts will be abolished too. From 1 April 2014 all NHS hospital and community trusts are required to become foundation trusts. Foundation trusts may enter into joint ventures with and distribute surpluses to for-profit companies; they can also raise commercial loans without restriction. The NHSCB and general practice consortiums will also have powers to form and invest in commercial companies. It is estimated that at least fifty trusts (hospitals and services) will not make foundation trust status and are likely to have to merge, will be closed or will be franchised out to the private sector.[12]

Provider regulation will be overseen by Monitor, which is charged with a duty to promote competition. Controversially, regulation by Monitor and the Care Quality Commission (CQC) will be chiefly through commercial licensing and contracting and limited by a duty of 'maximising the autonomy of individual commissioners and providers and minimising the obligations placed upon them'. Regulators are required not to impose 'unnecessary burdens' and regulation can be dispensed with as more providers enter the marketplace. The 'necessity' of public regulation can be challenged by corporations in the courts. Proposals by the European Commission to introduce such tests to health services created Europe-wide controversy in 2004 and had to be withdrawn because they were deemed to conflict with public health policies, such as controls over market access. However, conflict between competition policy and the Health Secretary's duty to promote a comprehensive service will be resolved not by Parliament but by Monitor, 'in the manner it considers best'.

Chapter 2 of the act introduces new competition duties that will allow remaining public controls over health services to be challenged by multinational companies and investors anywhere in the world. Trade rules outlaw public policies that prevent, restrict or distort competition in trade within the UK or the European Union, such as setting prices, instituting public subsidies for teaching and research, and designing controls to ensure fair distribution of resources. Rules on free movement of capital could undermine powers that the government proposes to reserve for protection of service continuity. The private health care company Circle, the first to take over a foundation trust, is already using competition rules to challenge a primary care trust's decision to restrict the volume and range of services under the commercial contracts for NHS elective surgery.

THE END OF UNIVERSAL HEALTH

In the absence of a ministerial responsibility it has become possible to blur the boundaries between free health care and chargeable care as they are for NHS continuing care and means-tested long-term care following the NHS and Community Care Act in 1990. NHS services are being made the responsibility of local authorities, which can charge for care. During the passage of the Health and Social Care Act last year the services to be transferred to local authorities included:[13]

- immunization, cancer and cardiovascular screening;
- mental health care;
- dental public health;
- public health;
- sexual health services;
- management of drug and alcohol addiction;
- emergency planning and health protection service;
- child health services.

The act also abolished rules making certain health services mandatory. The following services are no longer required by law to be provided free of charge:[14]

- services and facilities for pregnant women, women who are breast-feeding;
- services for both younger and older children;
- services for the prevention of illness;
- care of persons suffering from illness and their after-care;
- ambulance services;
- services for people with mental illness;
- dental public health services;
- sexual health services.

Under the new system, players in the health care market can choose the services they wish to provide and the patients for whom they provide them. The principle is not, as the Coalition Government repeatedly claimed, increased patient choice but increased *choice of patient*.

THE COMING AGE OF HEALTH CARE FOR PROFIT

The new and highly controversial rules governing procurement, competitive tendering and commercial contracting coupled with deregulation expand the possibilities for the private for-profit sector. Free of the responsibilities under which public bodies have to act, commercial firms can take on a larger health care role and greater control over resource use in the NHS. This is not an accident. The government is determined that commercial corporations, not doctors and other health professionals, will control health spending. Accordingly, more and more NHS services are being put out to tender to for-profit companies and taxpayer funds are being given to commercial corporations whilst publicly run health facilities are closed down.

As the Health and Social Care Act is now being implemented, corporations will immediately have more say in determining our entitlement to free health services. In future, no single organisation will be responsible for ensuring all of an area's health care, and it will no longer be clear who should be held accountable when things go wrong.

Our relationship with our doctor will change when for-profit companies run more services. As a patient we will no longer necessarily come first: how can we feel confident that our doctor is putting us first when he or she is a for-profit company employee?

Privatisation and marketisation have already increased in advance of the 2012 act. Some services, including those for the most vulnerable people in society, have been contracted out to for-profit companies such as Virgin and Serco Group, which have little or no experience in delivering health care. These companies have taken on services for children with mental health problems and physical disabilities in Devon,[15] and community nursing and health visitor services in Surrey[16] and Suffolk.[17]

Many NHS hospitals are owned and operated under the expensive Private Finance Initiative, creating serious financial problems for them and putting neighbouring hospitals and services at risk.[18] For-profit companies and investors now control GP practices and other local health services. According to the *Financial Times*, Virgin already earns around £200 million a year by running more than one hundred NHS services nationwide, including GP surgeries.[19] A private company registered in the Virgin Islands now manages the local hospital in Huntingdon, Hinchingbrooke NHS Trust.

MANUFACTURED DEFICITS

It is clear that the government is manufacturing a crisis, reducing the level of services and their quality, and shaking public confidence in the NHS. We are being encouraged to accept the principle that we will in future have to pay privately for services that were once free.

Malcolm Grant, formerly the provost of University College London and now the chair of NHS England, himself does not use the NHS and in the past has supported higher education tuition charges. In April 2013 he said: 'It's not my responsibility to introduce new charging systems but it's something which a future government will wish to reflect [on], unless the economy has picked up sufficiently, because we can anticipate demand for NHS services rising by about 4 to 5 per cent per annum'. But there is no justification for these claims.

Since 1948 politicians and the Treasury have been advocating greater use of charges in the NHS. Compare Grant's careless talk with the stand of Aneurin Bevan, the architect of the NHS who resigned over the principle of charges, or with the noble sentiments expressed by the 1979 Royal Commission on the NHS, which rejected charging: 'We can say clearly the NHS is not suffering from a mortal disease susceptible only to heroic surgery. Already the NHS has achieved a great deal and embodies aspirations and ideals of great value. The advances to be made – and which undoubtedly will be made – will be brought about by constant application and vigilance.'[20]

Similarly, the claims today that we can no longer afford the NHS are untrue. The NHS is not over budget. In 2012, in the midst of the debate over the health act, the NHS budget was underspent and £2 billion was returned to the Treasury.[21] Headline stories about hospital and other health service deficits only mean that resources are unfairly distributed, not that the NHS is unaffordable overall. Government claims that it is protecting the NHS budget are also untrue. According to the official watchdog, the Statistics Authority: 'expenditure on the NHS in real terms was lower in 2011–12 than it was in 2009–10'.[22]

The NHS is being run as if it is in a financial crisis but this crisis is of the government's making. Current plans for cutting NHS budgets, closing hospital beds and making thousands of vital NHS staff redundant are based on documents drawn up by management consultancy firms including the US firm McKinsey & Company.[23] The policy will lead to closure and hollowing out of public services, and the creation of opportunities for an expanded market for private provision and the introduction of user charges.

The policy is fuelling cuts, closures and mergers on a scale that is unparalleled:

Cuts and closures[24]
• In north-west London the government plans to cut 25% of beds, and throughout London at least 7 A&E departments will close, with further departments under threat. Up to 5,600 jobs in north-west London will be lost by 2015. Barnet and Chase Farm Hospitals NHS Trust is cutting 208 posts.
• In Merseyside 4,000 NHS jobs will go by 2014.
• In South Yorkshire Rotherham Hospital is set to lose 750 staff by 2015.
• In West Suffolk Serco is planning to cut 137 community health care jobs.
• In Devon and Exeter the Royal Devon and Exeter NHS Foundation Trust plans to cut 1,115 full-time equivalent posts between 2011 and 2014.
• In Greater Manchester there are plans to downgrade Trafford General Hospital's A&E to urgent care, and make cuts to intensive care, acute surgery and children's services. Maternity services have already closed. Salford Royal NHS Foundation Trust plans to cut 750 full-time posts by 2013. Bolton NHS trust is making 500 redundancies.
• In Warwickshire the George Eliot Hospital NHS Trust plans to cut the equivalent of 257 full-time staff between 2010 and 2014.
• In Cornwall Royal Hospital Truro proposed to cut 400 jobs in 2011.
• In Portsmouth Queen Alexandra Hospital cut 700 jobs and shut 3 wards in 2011.
• Across England 24 out of 30 NHS Direct call centres will close.
• Since the Coalition came to power in 2010 6,000 nursing posts have been cut.

Mergers

- Hospital mergers reduce services and increase waiting times and travel distances.

- Merger with North Tees was followed by closure of A&E in Hartlepool in August 2011.

- Merger of South London Trust is followed by recommendation of closure of Lewisham Hospital A&E.

- Merger of Queen Mary's Sidcup NHS Trust (QMS), Queen Elizabeth Hospital NHS Trust (QEH) and Bromley Hospitals NHS Trust (BHT) to create a single hospital on several sites in 2009 was followed by closure of Queen Mary's A&E and labour unit in 2010.

- Merger of Norfolk and Waveney and Suffolk mental health trusts was followed by cuts in beds for acute mental illness and community mental health teams.

- Barnet and Chase Farm Hospitals NHS Trust currently plans a merger that is likely to result in closure of A&E, maternity and paediatric services.

- Merger resulted in closure of Trafford General Maternity Unit in 2010 and A&E is threatened.

- Merger with Blackburn Hyndburn and Ribble Valley (BHRV) NHS Trust in 2003 was followed by closure of Burnley A&E in 2008 and the paediatric inpatient ward in 2010.

- Merger resulted in closure of Rochdale Infirmary, Greater Manchester A&E in 2011.

There is no evidence to support change on this scale or the unfair distribution of funds.[25]

Underpinning these cuts is the government's claims of poor

hospital performance and misleading use of statistics on hospital mortality rates and financial performance. The policy of attributing poor performance and deficits to individual hospitals – taken for granted today – is a dangerous one, as Treasury mandarin Sir Richard Clarke pointed out in 1964: 'In the dispersed services such as education and hospitals … units of administration are small, and their performance must be uneven. It is difficult to form a judgement about how efficient those relatively small independent units are, and how much scope there may be for saving, and by what management techniques and services this potential saving can be realised – without of course endangering the quality of local responsibility and flexibility to local circumstances which is fundamental to these services.'[26]

HOPE: REINSTATEMENT OF THE NHS

The Health and Social Care Act 2012 must be revoked because it removes the democratic and legal basis of the NHS and allows services to be closed and reconfigured on an unprecedented scale. The Coalition Government has no mandate for this act. We did not vote for the abolition of our NHS. Neither was it a part of the Coalition agreement. And unlike those citizens who reside in England, citizens of Scotland, Wales and Northern Ireland will continue to have an NHS – under the law.

In February 2013 Lord Owen, himself a former Health Minister, took up the challenge and tabled a private members' bill in the House of Lords that would reinstate the Secretary of State's duty to provide comprehensive health services:

> Some will say why go to all this trouble, if a Labour
> government wins more votes than the Conservatives

it will not be necessary. The answer to that question is that some of the changes which we are proposing in this short Bill amend both Labour and Conservative legislation, both the 2006 and the 2012 Acts of Parliament. It is also not enough to have a new government and a new Secretary of State for Health. The Health and Social Care Act of 2012 is drafted so that decision making is not controlled by the Secretary of State who only has severely limited powers of intervention. A Cabinet, let alone a Secretary of State does not change the law of the land merely by being elected – they have to legislate and there are many pressures on them for urgent legislation. A short Bill that has been discussed over a few years, championed in elections and won the support of the vast majority of people who work in the NHS, should be able to win the competition for legislative time. A government that seeks to act in advance of the legislation could well be repulsed, subjected to judicial review and challenged in the courts of law. This 2012 Act was especially drafted to take away the powers of the Secretary of State and vest huge power in the largest ever quasi, autonomous, non-governmental organisation or Quango, the NHS Commissioning Board. The commercial entities that will start from April 2013 in ever increasing numbers to marketise the NHS will not be ready purely because of a General Election, to acquiesce in the stopping of contractual negotiations. They will want to push ahead and get in under the wire. It is also very necessary to make crystal clear that it is very unlikely that such commercial organisations could guarantee on tendering for an ever increasing flow of NHS contracts after the next General Election.[27]

His bill restores the legal and democratic basis of the NHS and the citizens' rights to hold the Secretary of State to ultimate account. It will restore the Secretary of State's duty to provide the NHS in England and gives him or her ministerial powers of direction and planning in order that the duty can be properly discharged.

Specifically, the Owen bill, the NHS (Amended Duties and Powers) Bill 2013, will:[28]

- reinstate the Secretary of State's duty to provide health services that was formerly contained within Sections 1 and 3 of the National Health Service Act 2006;
- subject all NHS bodies and bodies providing services for the NHS to ministerial direction;
- repeal the duty of autonomy and restore sufficient ministerial control over provision consistent with the Secretary of State's overarching duty to provide health services to the whole of England;
- give Monitor an objective, so that its purpose is to help deliver the NHS.

England is not alone in its assault on universal health care. Many European countries are following suit, both reducing health service budgets and abolishing their national health services as part of the response to their economic crisis. In 2012 Portugal raised user charges for health care by €150 million. In 2013 charges will be raised by another €50 million. Between 2011 and 2012 Greece increased user fees and cut the country's health budget by €1.4 billion. The Czech Republic cut their budget by 30 per cent. At the end of last year Spain implemented a royal decree to repeal overnight its universal health care law and major reductions in health spending and structural market reforms have been agreed in Ireland, Ukraine,

Latvia, Romania, Hungary, Iceland, the Czech Republic, France, the Netherlands and Austria. In all these cases, as in England, households are being forced to take on more of the financial risks of illness.

Meanwhile, in the low- and middle-income countries of the world, international aid is increasingly aligned with policies that rely on households continuing to pay for health care. These policies set aside the World Health Organisation's long-standing commitment to elimination of co-payments: an era of safety nets in which tax-financed care is limited to the indigent has replaced the era of universal access. The results can only be diminished services for the poor and not-so-poor in a climate of growing injustice.

Proponents of the argument that tax-financed or 'free' health care is a privilege we can no longer afford are unable to explain why universal health care was instituted when the world's economy was very much smaller than it is today. If the UK could create an NHS when the country was literally bankrupt, why in England can the government not sustain the NHS today?

The answer of course is political not financial. Scotland, Wales and Northern Ireland still have an NHS and have thus far resisted market pressure despite the cuts. The market-driven changes in England are the culmination of a transition from public to private responsibility and market dogma has penetrated, only to abolish an institution that has defined us in our own eyes and internationally. By removing the mandate on government to provide a comprehensive health service throughout England, the Health and Social Care Act 2012 is the ultimate act of vandalism in this long funereal recessional from universality.

Nye Bevan said of the NHS that it 'will last as long as there are folk left with the faith to fight for it'. The wanton destruction of our universal public health care system is a catastrophe. It is also an act of tyranny. The NHS in England must be re-established.

Our response must be political.

8

STOP PRESS: THE FINAL BETRAYAL

David Wrigley and Jacky Davis

In February 2012, when his bill was in trouble, Andrew Lansley wrote to English GPs promising 'it is a fundamental principle of the bill that you as commissioners ... should decide when and how competition should be used'.[1] As has been seen, his reassurance was used to gain urgently needed support for the bill.

When secondary legislation, including section 75[2] of the Health and Social Care Act 2012, which dealt with contracts and competition, was quietly laid in Parliament on 11 February 2013, it didn't at first attract much attention, and the Coalition undoubtedly hoped it would remain that way. However, campaigners soon woke up to the fact that something was afoot. On 19 February an article appeared online, written by medical academic Dr Lucy Reynolds and journalist Nicola Cutcher, entitled 'The NHS as we know it needs a prayer'.[3] The piece addressed the threats concealed in section 75. As Dr Reynolds said in an illuminating interview, 'the Health and Social Care Act was an airplane with no jet engines and the regulations issued in February 2013 are the jet engines that allow the privatisation of the NHS to go ahead.'[4]

Some Lib Dem peers were unhappy and sought an urgent meeting with Earl Howe, who was leading on health for the Coalition Government in the House of Lords. Baroness Williams, Lady Jolly and Lord Clement Jones had concerns about the original wording of the enabling legislation and asked for amendments to it. The wording was altered and Baroness Williams claimed in Hansard[5] that she and her colleagues were responsible for the rewriting of the regulations. Yet again the Lib Dems were posing as saviours of the NHS, but their subsequent actions in the voting lobby would show where their true loyalties lay.

The wording may have been altered but, as with the original bill during the listening pause, it made no substantive difference. As NHS campaigner Caroline Malloy of openDemocracy tweeted: 'same meat, different gravy'.[6] The new regulations stated that clinical commissioning groups (CCGs) would be required to put services out to tender unless they could be sure that only one provider was able to offer the service. This was interpreted by many as creating a potential field day for lawyers. CCGs, on their meagre budgets, would never be able to demonstrate beyond legal challenge that only one provider was able to offer any service. They would always have to take the safe route of going out to tender.

The proposed legislation thus constituted a blatant breach of Lansley's promise that CCGs could choose when and with whom to commission. The BMA General Practitioners Committee overwhelmingly condemned it on 21 March 2013. After weeks of characteristic self-doubt and delay, and with only five days to go before the Lords debate that was scheduled, the BMA leadership also joined the opponents of section 75 and on 18 April published a briefing on their newfound opposition.[7]

Other organisations also expressed major concerns, but once again the voice of the majority of the medical royal colleges was barely audible. One highly decorated president wrote to Dr David Wrigley, who had organised a second 'Call on your College' campaign, that he had – 'received adequate reassurances from Lord Howe and Lansley that there was no desire to increase privatisation of clinical services'. This was rather like having reassurances from the Pied Piper of Hamelin that it was safe to leave your children with him.

The political opposition was led by Labour's Lord Hunt, who 'laid a prayer' to force a debate on the legislation in the House of Lords, which took place on 24 April. Lord Hunt opened by saying, 'I believe that the regulations are part of the Government's drive to shift the culture of the NHS from a public service into a public marketplace'. [8] Lord Howe then tried to reassure the House: 'there is no government agenda to privatise NHS services'.[9]

Baroness Williams was presumably feeling guilty following her support for the Health and Social Care Act 2012. She complained: 'I got a bit fed up with being constantly described as either a turncoat or a traitor' but apparently not that fed up, as she added, 'I am afraid we cannot go back; we are where we are'.[10] And with that she voted with the rest of the Lib Dem peers who were present, who had been placed under a three-line whip by the leadership to vote with their Conservative colleagues in the Coalition. Yet again the Lib Dems had co-operated in pushing through legislation that would damage the NHS through increased privatisation.

A number of the peers present had interests in private health care companies, and would thus potentially benefit financially from the passage of the legislation. Lord Norman Warner, the only Labour peer to break ranks[11] started his speech by declaring his registered interest as an adviser to two companies and went on to vote with the Coalition. There were calls for his expulsion from the Labour party for his treachery.

Only fifty-one per cent of Labour peers were present for the debate. The attempt to stop the regulations was lost by 254 votes to 146.

This was the final nail in the coffin of the publicly-provided NHS. Lord Owen caught the mood of many when he said, 'I warn this house: do not think that this is a minor step ... tonight I feel one feeling only: overwhelming sadness'.

Afterword

WHAT YOU CAN DO
TO SAVE THE NHS

Jacky Davis and Raymond Tallis

*Philosophers have hitherto described the world. The
point, however, is to change it.*

Karl Marx

*Describe the challenges by all means but don't
confuse analysis with action. The one must lead to the
other if it is to be useful.*

Michael Foot

The impending destruction of the National Health Service has
been a long time in the making, as will be clear from the foregoing
pages. Andrew Lansley's Health and Social Care Act did not come

out of the blue. It had taken thirty years of preparation, during which successive administrations undermined the values and assumptions that had made the NHS possible while at the same time seeming to uphold them. The story told in these chapters is one of barefaced lying and hypocrisy; of a contempt for the democratic process within national and local politics, and within professional bodies; undeclared conflicts of interest that would make Transparency International blush; and failures within the media to expose the politicians' real agenda for the NHS and to inform its audience about a matter of such supreme importance.

Anyone who cares for the NHS – that is to say, for the health and well-being of the people of this country – needs to appreciate that, while it is not too late to save the NHS from destruction by what Polly Toynbee has described as 'ideologically propelled vandalism', it will not be easy. This will be evident from the extraordinary, indeed outrageous, events described in the chapters of this book.

Several key lessons should inform any campaign to mitigate the consequences of Lansley's act and the policies of Labour and Tory administrations that prepared the ground for it:

1. Politicians are prepared to lie to the population at large, to those who vote for them, and to the activists within their own parties. Being caught lying, once fatal for a political career, will be dealt with by more lies.

2. Many organisations and individuals who have been involved in developing NHS policy and who are cheerleaders for the 'reforms' that threaten the future of the NHS have strong pecuniary interests in 'marketising' health care.[1] They will hardly be amenable to reasoned concerns

about the impact of the act. The best that can be hoped for is that they will take their money and run.

3. The leaders of professional bodies – supposedly representing the views of their membership and the interests of patients – may pay scant regard to the democratic process and may have undeclared reasons for doing so.

4. Many of the changes that will impinge directly on patient care are not always easy to understand. It takes persistence to see through the rhetoric that conceals the real intent of 'reforms'. In addition, the act runs alongside the target for £20 billion of cuts ('efficiency savings') by June 2015. This is already resulting in the 'reconfiguration' of hospital services, with cutbacks and closures of A&E, beds and whole hospitals. These plans are also dressed up in bland, vague language and require close reading to identify what's missing, and therefore what the real proposals are.

5. Information about what has happened, what is happening, and what is about to happen will be difficult to obtain. Considerations of 'commercial confidentiality' will trump any Freedom of Information requests.

6. The media, who, with a few honourable exceptions, failed in their duty to question, inform and warn their audiences of the nature of the act and who did not hold the policymakers and their backers to account, may regard the NHS 'reforms' as yesterday's news.

7. What is more, this view may be shared even by those who were opposed to Lansley's bill from the start. Surely, it may be argued, it is too late. As Tony Blair might say, 'We are where we are. It is time to move on.'

But there are many things we can do if we are well informed and well organised, and the fight to reclaim our NHS will continue as long as there are people who care for it and what it stands for.

GENERAL STRATEGY

Political pressure

We must make it clear to Coalition Government politicians of both Houses that we will not forgive or forget their profoundly anti-democratic behaviour. There are over a million people working in the NHS. Our votes and those of our friends and families can be used to hold to account the politicians responsible for its betrayal. We must also hold Labour to their public promises to reverse the legislation when they are back in power. They must promise to adopt Lord Owen's bill.

There is also a new political party, the National Health Action Party, which is dedicated to reclaiming and restoring a publicly funded, publicly delivered and publicly accountable NHS, which will be standing candidates at the next election. The betrayal of the NHS and its consequences will be an important issue at the next election. We must keep it in the spotlight until then.

Campaigns

Many people have now woken up to the dangers of the act and want to actively campaign. You can join established campaigning organisations such as Keep Our NHS Public, the NHS Support Federation and 38 Degrees. Some have formed special interest groups – public health doctors, medical students and patients' groups have all organised to add their voices and particular knowledge to the growing protest. In addition, there are many groups being set up around the country in response to local cuts and closures, which usually work both around local threats and in conjunction with national campaigns. Time and money are needed to campaign effectively and those who are able should consider giving whichever they can.

While all these local and national organisations can and do work in parallel, they are also starting to join forces. We are already seeing joint conferences, to decide the way ahead for the forces of opposition, and it must be made clear to politicians that we do not consider that the fight is over.

Tracking the changes

We will have to work together to monitor the changes to the NHS now that the act is taking effect. As already noted, it will be increasingly difficult to know what is going on, as the service fragments and financial dealings and patient outcomes are lost behind a convenient curtain of 'commercial confidentiality'. It is essential that we keep track of the real effects of the act if we are to show that we were right about its dangers.

The NHS Support Federation already have a site to track privatisation:

http://www.nhscampaign.org/NHS-reforms/privatisation/track-ing-privatisation.html.

Unite are asking for reports of cuts and closures: http://www.unitetheunion.org/how-we-help/list-of-sectors/healthsector/healthsectorcampaigns/unite4ournhs/saveournhsshareyourstory.

The price of knowledge is eternal vigilance. The Coalition certainly won't be telling us about the problems that arise; it will be our responsibility to monitor them. The stories that have made headlines, for example of Serco 'fiddling the books' over its out-of-hours service,[2] have come to light via local MPs and the press. Social media such as Twitter are particularly useful to campaigners for sharing and disseminating this sort of information and most campaigning organisations have a Twitter presence.

Holding leaders to account

We need an urgent inquest into the abysmal failure of professional 'leadership' in the face of the bill. Most of the leaders of the professions moved to opposition only after internal struggles and grass-roots organisation, achieved via unofficial online polls, through social networking sites, and with calls for emergency general meetings.

With few exceptions – most notably the Royal College of General Practitioners – the behaviour of the leadership of the professional bodies was strikingly undemocratic, myopic and supine. The leaders of the professions failed to represent their members, and their failure first to understand and then to act effectively against the bill still remains to be explained. They must be held to account for this and the whole structure of professional representation would benefit from a critical examination.

Members and fellows of such bodies should remind the leadership of their failure to protect the interests of patients and insist that, given that the situation is remediable, they should be prepared to voice their opposition. Specifically, campaigners should:

1. hold the leadership to account at major meetings such as the BMA annual representative meeting;

2. support members of decision-making bodies who genuinely care for the NHS and will fight for its future.

As a further example of what might be done, the president of the Royal College of Physicians (RCP) has already been challenged for the post on the basis of the RCP's poor showing during the passage of the bill.[3] This is such an unusual and important development that *The Lancet* gave it front-page billing and it came close to ejecting the incumbent.[4]

Look ahead

It is easy to be so taken up with fire-fighting immediate problems that we overlook the big picture. It is particularly important for campaigning health policy analysts and those with legal knowledge to keep an eye on what is in the pipeline. At the time of writing, the looming problem is the EU/US trade agreement that threatens to 'harmonise' the NHS. When applied to health, this means that the whole emphasis of health care changes. The rights of transnational corporations become the priority and health becomes primarily a trade issue.[5]

PRACTICAL STEPS

Get involved with a local NHS campaign group. This could be a group affiliated to a national campaign such as Keep Our NHS Public (KONP) or 38 Degrees, or a local campaign focused on local issues. The issue that is most often at the centre of local campaigns is the threat of closures or severe cutbacks in local services: don't miss the chance to link up with these movements – those involved will often be receptive to explanations and discussion of the wider agenda behind the cuts.

If there isn't a local campaign group, think about forming one, to bring together individuals who are opposed to, or at least concerned about, the implications of the act. The national office of KONP can help you do this, with campaign materials and a speaker for your first meeting. Campaign materials can be found at: http://www.keepournhspublic.com/campaignresources.php.

Many other organisations also have guidance about how to campaign, for instance the NHS Support Federation has a lot of helpful information: http://www.nhscampaign.org.uk/new_campaign_guide/fed_campaign_guide.html#2.

On the local level, here are some specific actions you can take:

Action 1   Attend clinical commissioning group (CCG) board meetings. Ask your CCGs to adopt a pro-NHS code, and to publish all their board papers, or explain where proposals are being withheld from public view. Identify the members of CCG boards and any conflicts of interest they may have and use them as reasons for closer scrutiny of decisions that are made.

Action 2   Get involved in the patient participation group (PPG) at your GP's surgery. If there isn't one, ask if you can set one up.

Action 3   Gather evidence from patients of withdrawal or rationing of services.

Action 4   Sign and distribute the Keep Our NHS Public postcard that patients can give to their GPs expressing their preference, where possible, to be treated by public not private providers. (A sample postcard is available at: http://www.kee-pournhspublic.com/campaignresources.php.)

Action 5   Identify and engage with sympathetic local GPs who may let you distribute campaign material in their surgeries.

Action 6   Find out and monitor proposed changes to your local services. Challenge any attempt to change – reconfigure, reduce, withdraw – services on anything other than sound clinical grounds. Proposals should be tied to clear, specific, costed and timetabled plans to replace threatened services and establish a new and improved model of care *before* any closures take place. Good intentions and fine words are not enough to justify closing actual services in your community.

Action 7   Find out which services are being outsourced to the private sector in your area. Monitor the tendering processes and the awarding of contracts. Demand that the processes should be transparent. Look into the background of firms whose tenders are successful. Examine the terms and conditions and the 'get-out' clauses.

Action 8   Help to mobilise public opinion with events, petitions, marches and other protests. Most people are more easily engaged over local issues such as cuts and closures of local services – so when you discover that a cut is being proposed, rally people to fight it.

Action 9   Identify people in your area who are media savvy and who are prepared to comment to the press and appear on local/national TV and radio about health issues. Others may be willing to write letters to local papers and broadcasters. Cultivate, and keep informed, local journalists who are willing to report on and follow up issues.

Action 10   Write regularly – individually or collectively – to local MPs, irrespective of party. Ask MPs to attend and speak at local meetings, and to justify their position if pro 'reforms'. They know this will be an issue at the next election. Pressurise Labour councils to speak up against privatisation of the services in their locality.

On the national level, consider getting involved in the following ways:

Action 1   If you have joined or set up a local group, contact the national organisations working on the NHS campaign – even if your group is set to campaign on local issues. This will help to convey powerfully that the mandate is for the NHS, not against it.

Action 2   Attend national conferences, participate in national marches and other forms of protest.

The more people who are seen standing up for the NHS, the more likely that the politicans and the media will listen.

Action 3   Be aware – and make others aware – that the most toxic elements of Lansley's reforms can be repealed without yet another expensive, disruptive reorganisation.

Action 4   Directly support Lord Owen's bill (see Appendix 1 and 2 for the text and explanatory notes) using petitions, the press, and your local political parties.

Action 5   Obtain reassurances from any politician for whom you are intending to vote or canvas in 2015 that they will support an amendment of the act. Even Lib Dems and Tories may be for the turning. Warn them that they will be held to their promises and that traditional levels of mendacity will not be tolerated. If there is a main party candidate in favour of amending the act, support him or her. If not, then support the candidates for the National Health Action Party.

Both campaigning groups and individuals can get involved in the formal structures for influencing the NHS and holding those who run it to account:

Action 1   Apply to become a member of your local hospital (foundation trust). Stand for election to become a governor or non-executive director of the board. Get together with like-minded people to stand on a platform of defence of the NHS and against expansion of private medicine.

Action 2   Healthwatch is designed to be toothless,[6] but it is worth considering getting involved in order to be able to 'rock the boat' from inside, reveal its limitations and lack of independence and discredit the 'reforms' they are part of.

Action 3   Talk to those inside the NHS who may be able to give important information off the record. Question the assumptions – such as the so-called 'Nicholson challenge' to save £20 billion – to justify cuts and reorganisations.

Action 4   Call on local councils to use their new power to open up Health and Wellbeing boards. Make them public platforms to debate local health policy and provision by co-opting or inviting participation of local pensioners, community organisations, TUC, health unions and professional bodies. The boards should meet in public, publicise their discussions and call local NHS managers to account. Stand for election to them, or seek to be co-opted.

Action 5   Attend local Health Scrutiny and Oversight committees, submit information to them, draw their attention to cutbacks, privatisation and other issues of local concern.

Action 6   Identify members of the Local Authority Health Overview and Scrutiny Committee and be prepared to raise issues with individual councillors. Identify membership of local area teams and attend their public meetings. Question their decisions if they do not seem clearly driven by patients' needs.

Envoi

Andrew Lansley's wrecking ball is a symptom of a deep corruption in British politics: his act would not have entered the statute book without the subversion of the democratic process and the collusion of many who should have opposed it. Decisions that will have an incalculable adverse effect on the health and well-being of the majority and will benefit a few have been taken largely out of sight. Legitimate government has been bypassed and we need to claim it back.

But the NHS remains the most cherished institution in the country, more so even than the monarchy,[7] and sitting back and watching it being torn apart is not an option. This is a fight worth fighting and one that we cannot afford to lose. At stake is the NHS itself. The NHS is embarked on a course that could end with the provision of skid row services for all except the minority who can afford expensive private insurance premiums – poor services for poor people.

David Cameron recently quoted Tony Blair's advice on reform: '[Reform] comes about and within a short amount of time, it is as if it has always been so. The opposition is inevitable, but it's rarely unbeatable.'[8]

In response we should offer him the words of Professor Harry Keen, indefatigable fighter for the NHS: 'The government intends to hold the NHS under water until the bubbles stop rising. But the bubbles will never stop rising.'

Further Resources

NATIONAL CAMPAIGNS ON THE NHS

- **Keep Our NHS Public (KONP)** – runs a national campaign as well as local groups across England. Campaigns for a publicly funded, publicly delivered and publicly accountable NHS.
  W www.keepournhspublic.com; T @keepnhspublic
- **London Health Emergency (LHE)** – campaigning against cuts, closures and the privatisation of the NHS since 1983.
  W http://www.healthemergency.org.uk; T @JohnRLister
- **NHS Support Federation** – an independent pressure group that campaigns to protect and improve the NHS, true to its founding principles.
  W http://www.nhscampaign.org; T @nhs_supporters
- **National Health Action Party (NHAP)** – campaigning for a publicly funded, publicly delivered and publicly account-able NHS.
  W http://www.nationalhealthaction.org.uk; T @NHAparty

ALLIED ORGANISATIONS

- **Centre for Health and the Public Interest** – a new independ-ent health think tank.
  W http://chpi.org.uk; T @CHPIthinktank

- **Medsin** – student network and registered charity tackling global and local health inequalities through education, advocacy and community action.
  W http://www.medsin.org/; **T** @medsinuk
- **NHS Consultants' Association** – organisation of hospital doctors who support the NHS and campaign to end market-based policies.
  W http://www.nhsca.org.uk/
- **openDemocracy** – 'free thinking for the world'. Running 'OurNHS', a new three-year project dedicated to reinstating a genuine National Health Service in England.
  W http://www.opendemocracy.net/ournhs/about;
  T @OurNHS_oD
- **Spinwatch** – works for lobbying transparency, promotes greater understanding of the role of PR and propaganda.
  W http://www.spinwatch.org/; **T** @Spinwatch
- **38 Degrees** – online organisation that brings people together to take action on the issues 'that matter to you and bring about real change'.
  W http://www.38degrees.org.uk/; **T** @38_degrees

FURTHER READING AND WATCHING

- *Health Policy Reform: Global Health versus Private Profit* by John Lister (Libri Publishing, 2013).
- *NHS plc: The Privatisation of Our Health Care* by Allyson M. Pollock (Verso Books, 2004).
- *The Plot Against the NHS* by Colin Leys and Stewart Player (Merlin Press, 2011).
- *Privatizing the World: A Study of International Privatization in Theory and Practice* by Oliver Letwin (Cengage Learning EMEA, 1988).

- 'The NHS and the section 75 regulations: Where next?' by Bob Hudson, *Guardian* healthcare network, 30 April 2012, http://www.guardian.co.uk/healthcare-network/2013/apr/30/nhs-section-75-regulations-where-next. This helpful article covers some additional actions that can be taken by opponents of the health care reforms.
- *Conflicts of Interest and NHS Privatisation*, video by the National Health Action Party, http://www.spinwatch.org/index.php/component/k2/item/5441-conflicts-of-interest-and-the-privatisation-of-the-nhs.
- *Take a Tour of Lansley's Private Healthcare Supporters*, video by Spinwatch, http://www.spinwatch.org/index.php/component/k2/item/5336-take-a-tour-of-Lansleys-private-health-care-supporters.
- *The Spirit of '45*, a film by Ken Loach, for screenings and availability see http://www.thespiritof45.com.

Text Of Lord Owen's

Amendments

The National Health Service (Amended Duties and Powers) Bill

A

BILL

TO

Re-establish the Secretary of State's legal duty as to the National Health Service in England, QUANGOS and related bodies.

BE IT ENACTED by the Queen's most Excellent Majesty, by and with the advice and consent of the Lords Spiritual and Temporal, and Commons, in this present

Parliament assembled, and by the authority of the same, as follows:—

1. Secretary of State's duties to promote and provide a comprehensive and integrated health service

For section 1 of the National Health Service Act 2006 (Secretary of State's duty to promote comprehensive health service) substitute:

1. Secretary of State's duty as to the health service

(1) It shall be the duty of the Secretary of State to promote in England a comprehensive and integrated health service designed to secure improvement –

    (a) in the physical and mental health of the people of England, and

    (b) in the prevention, diagnosis and treatment of illness, and for that purpose to provide or secure the effective provision of services in accordance with this Act.

(2) The services so provided must be free of charge except in so far as the making and recovery of charges is expressly provided for by or under any enactment, whenever passed.

(3) The services provided pursuant to this Act and to the Health and Social Care Act 2012, howsoever or by whomsoever provided, secured or arranged, shall be deemed to be provided in furtherance of the duty to provide or secure effective provision of services under subsection (1)."

2. Abolition of the duties of autonomy

Section 1D and section 13F of the National Health Service Act 2006 (duties as to promoting autonomy) are repealed.

3. Concurrent duty of and commissioning by the NHS Commissioning Board

(1) Section 1H(2) of the National Health Service Act 2006 is repealed.

(2) In section 1H(3) of that Act, for "For the purpose of discharging that duty," substitute "For the purpose of

furthering the duty of the Secretary of State under section 1(1),".

4. Secretary of State's duty as to provision of certain services

(1) Section 3 of the National Health Service Act 2006 is amended as follows.

(2) Before subsection (1) insert—

"(Z1) The Secretary of State must provide or secure the effective provision throughout England, to such extent as he considers necessary to meet all reasonable requirements, the accommodation, services and facilities set out in subsection (1)(a)-(f)."

(3) In subsection (1), before "A", insert "For that purpose,".

5. Power of directions to QUANGOs and other bodies

(1) The Secretary of State may direct any of the bodies mentioned in subsection (2) to exercise any of his functions relating to the health service which are specified in the directions, and may also give directions to any such body about its exercise of any functions or about its provision of services under arrangements referred to in subsection 2(h).

(2) The bodies are—

(a) the National Health Service Commissioning Board

(b) a clinical commissioning group,

(c) a Special Health Authority,

(d) an NHS trust,

(e) an NHS foundation trust,

(f) the National Institute for Health and Care Excellence,

(g) the Health and Social Care Information Centre, and

(h) any other body or person providing services in pursuance of arrangements made—

      (i) by the Secretary of State under section 12,

      (ii) by the Board or a clinical commissioning group under section 3, 3A, 3B or 4 or Schedule 1,

      (iii) by a local authority for the purpose of the exercise of its functions under or by virtue of section 2B or 6C(1) or Schedule 1, or

      (iv) by the Board, a clinical commissioning group or a local authority by virtue of section 7A of the National Health Service Act 2006.

(3) In exercising his power under subsection (1), the Secretary of State must have regard to the desirability, so far as consistent with the interests of the health service and relevant to the exercise of the power in all the circumstances—

  (a) of protecting and promoting the health of patients and the public;

  (b) of any of the bodies mentioned in subsection (2) being free, in exercising its functions or providing services in accordance with its duties and powers, to do so in the manner that it considers best calculated to promote the comprehensive and integrated service referred to in section 1(1) of the National Health Service Act 2006; and

  (c) of ensuring cooperation between the bodies mentioned in subsection (2) in the exercise of their functions or provision of services.

(4) If, in having regard to the desirability of the matters referred to in subsection (3) the Secretary of State considers that there is a conflict between those matters and the discharge of his duties under section 1 of the National Health Service Act 2006, he must give priority to the duties under that section.

6. Monitor

(1) The Health and Social Care Act 2012 is amended as follows.

(2) After section 61 insert—

61A Monitor's objective

(1) The objective of Monitor is to contribute to the achievement of a comprehensive and integrated health service in England through the exercise of its functions.

(2) In exercising its main duty and other functions Monitor must act in accordance with that objective and in a manner consistent with the performance by the Secretary of State of his duties contained in sections 1 and 3 of the National Health Service Act 2006.

(3) Section 62(9) is repealed.

7. Interpretation

Expressions used in this Act which are also used in the National Health Service Act 2006 and in the Health and Social Care Act 2012 shall have the same meanings as the meanings given to those expressions under those Acts.

8. Short title, commencement and extent

(1) This Act may be cited as the National Health Service (Amended Duties and Powers) Act 2013.

(2) This Act shall come into force on the day on which it is passed.

(3) This Act extends to England.

Appendix 2

National Health Service
(Amended Duties and Powers) Bill

Explanatory Notes

These explanatory notes relate to the National Health Service (Amended Duties and Powers) Bill. They have been prepared in order to assist the reader of the bill and to help inform debate on it. They do not form part of the bill and have not been endorsed by Parliament.

The notes need to be read in conjunction with the bill. They are not, and are not meant to be, a comprehensive description of the bill. So where a clause or part of a clause does not seem to require any explanation or comment, none is given.

COMMENTARY ON CLAUSES

Clause 1 – Secretary of State's duties to promote and provide a comprehensive and integrated health service

3. This Clause, in conjunction with Clause 4, would reinstate the Secretary of State's legal duty to provide the NHS in England. It would do so by effectively repealing the

abolition of that duty as a result of section 1 of the Health and Social Care Act 2012, and by reproducing the corresponding provision applying in Scotland, namely section 1(1) of the National Health Service (Scotland) Act 1978.

4. Reproducing that provision would also mean that the duty would be to promote a comprehensive and integrated service. Including an integrated service within the government's fundamental duty would cohere with and provide a central basis for the various integration duties imposed by the 2012 act on the NHS Commissioning Board (the Board) (s.13N), on clinical commissioning groups (CCGs) (s.14Z1), on Monitor (s.62(4) and s.96), and on Health and Wellbeing Boards (s.195), as well as for the power given to local authorities and CCGs to make a statement about integration in the joint health and wellbeing strategy (s.193). In this way, re-establishing the Secretary of State's duties and powers to the NHS in England could be done – and strengthened as a response to the integration provisions of the 2012 act – without further reorganization.

5. The Clause would also strengthen the duty in England by requiring the Secretary of State to provide or secure the effective provision of services. This requirement was contained in the National Health Service acts of 1946 and 1977, but was removed in the National Health Service Act 2006. The 2006 act also de-coupled the duty to provide from the duty to promote, and this Clause would return both duties to the same subsection, in line with the 1946 and 1977 acts and, in Scotland, the 1978 act.

6. The title of section 1 of the 2006 act ("Secretary of State's duty to promote health service") would revert to the title of section 1 of the National Health Service Act 1977,

which made no distinction between the connected duties of promotion and provision.

7. Subsection (3) clarifies that the services provided under the 2006 act or under the 2012 act, whether directly or indirectly, would be so provided in furtherance of the Secretary of State's duty. These would include services provided as a result of arrangements made by the Board, CCGs and local authorities.

Clause 2 – Abolition of the duties of autonomy

8. This clause would repeal the two sections inserted into the 2006 act which require the Secretary of State and the NHS Commissioning Board, respectively, to have regard to the desirability of securing, so far as consistent with the interests of the health service, that any other person exercising functions in relation to the health service or providing services for its purposes is free to exercise those functions or provide those services in the manner that it considers most appropriate, and that unnecessary burdens are not imposed on any such person. These duties are incompatible with a national health service which the Secretary of State would, under this bill, again have the duty to provide.

9. However, certain elements of section 1D of the 2006 act in relation to the Secretary of State's power of directions would be retained under Clause 5(3) and (4) of the bill.

Clause 3 – Concurrent duty of and commissioning by the NHS Commissioning Board

10. Clause 3(1) would repeal section 1H(2) of the 2006 act, inserted by section 9 of the 2012 act, which subjects the Board to the duty under section 1(1) of the 2006 act concurrently with the Secretary of State (except in relation to

the public health functions of the Secretary of State and of local authorities).

11. That repeal requires an amendment to the opening words of section 1H(3) of the 2006 act, and this would be effected by Clause 3(2) which would make clear that the Board's commissioning functions are for the purpose of furthering the Secretary of State's duty under section 1(1) of that act.

Clause 4 – Secretary of State's duty as to provision of certain services

12. This clause would reinstate the duty of the Secretary of State to provide hospital accommodation, services and facilities as specified in section 3(1) of the 2006 act, and would extend it to include the duty, in the alternative, to secure their effective provision. This extension reflects the wording of section 1(1), and acknowledges that the government itself will not usually be providing services directly.

13. Because the focus of the bill is to re-establish the Secretary of State's duties without a further reorganisation, the 2012 act's transfer of this duty to each CCG (and, in the process, modifying it to a duty to arrange provision) would remain, but would be amended in order to make clear that a CCG's duty was for the purpose of implementing the Secretary of State's prior duty.

14. If the Secretary of State did not consider that implementation by CCGs of their individual duties was resulting in the provision of hospital accommodation, services and facilities as specified which he or she considered necessary to meet all reasonable requirements throughout England, the Secretary of State would be able to issue directions under clause 5.

15. The power could be exercised, for example, if implementation of the 2012 act risked putting the Secretary of State in breach of his duties under sections 1(1) and 3 (as modified by this bill). For example, regulations can be made under the 2012 act to exclude people from services (section 3(1D)), and only emergency care need be provided for everybody (pursuant to section 3(1C)). These new provisions were part of the shift effected by that act, away from the Secretary of State's area-based responsibility under s.3(1) ("throughout England") – subsequently delegated to primary care trusts established by order with responsibilities based on electoral wards – to list-based responsibilities of CCGs ("persons for whom a CCG is responsible"). If this shift were to result in everybody in England not being provided for, directions to one or more CCG under clause 5, for example, would be able to rectify the situation, and could require addressing the approach to the resource allocation formula.

Clause 5 – Power of directions to QUANGOs and other bodies

16. This Clause would give the Secretary of State a general power of giving directions to those quasi-autonomous non-governmental organisations (QUANGOs) and other bodies with health service functions and contracts who may be given emergency directions under section 253 of the 2006 act (as amended by section 47 of the 2012 act). This general power would be additional to other powers given to the Secretary of State by the 2012 act to give directions in other specific circumstances (for example, to direct the Board to exercise any of his or her functions relating to the provision of primary medical services, or to require

a clinical commissioning group to use specified banking facilities).

17. Clause 5(3) would seek to address concerns that the power of directions might be used in particular circumstances to impose an undesirable form of centralised control. It would therefore require the Secretary of State, before issuing relevant directions, to have regard to the desirability of, firstly, protecting and promoting the health of patients and the public. Such protection and promotion is an underlying purpose motivating establishment of the NHS, and is, for example, one of the key responsibilities of Good Medical Practice for doctors registered with the General Medical Council.

18. Secondly, regard would have to be had to the desirability of the QUANGOs and other bodies receiving directions being free to perform their functions in the manner that they consider best calculated to promote the comprehensive and integrated health service. This requirement is based on part of the duty of autonomy that was introduced in the 2012 act, with modifications to its precise terms and the circumstances in which the duty would arise. It could arise, for example, in situations envisaged by the Medical Innovation Bill where it might be desirable to support responsible innovation in cases where evidence to support particular courses of treatment or management is unavailable or uncertain.

19. Thirdly, under clause 5(3)(b) regard would also have to be had to the desirability of ensuring cooperation among the same bodies.

20. Clause 5(4) would preserve the purpose of section 1D(2) of the 2012 act, namely to preserve the precedence and priority of the duties to promote and provide under section 1.

Clause 6 – Monitor

21. Currently, there is no objective underpinning Monitor's powers and duties – unlike Ofgem, for example. This clause would make clear that the end to which its functions under the Health and Social Care Act 2012 must be directed is the comprehensive and integrated health service that it is the Secretary of State's duty to promote and provide under the National Health Service Act 2006.

22. This Clause would also – by inserting into the 2012 act a new section 61A(2) and by repealing section 62(9) – reinstate the duty of Monitor to act consistently with the Secretary of State's duties to promote and provide. Parliament had imposed that duty on Monitor both in section 32 of the 2006 act and in section 3 of the Health and Social Care (Community Health and Standards) Act 2003 (although in those enactments Monitor's duty also extended to acting consistently with the Secretary of State's duty in relation to university clinical teaching and research). The 2012 act, in section 62(9), only imposed a duty on Monitor in relation to the duty to promote under section 1(1) of the 2006 act, hence its proposed repeal under this clause.

Notes

Introduction

1 HM Government (2010), 'The Coalition: our programme for government', 19 May.

2 A recent estimate that it will cost £4 billion was cited in Nicholas Timmins's indispensable 2012 account of the passage of the Health and Social Care Act, *Never Again?: The Story of the Health and Social Care Act 2012 -- A Study in Coalition Government and Policy* (London: The King's Fund and Institute for Government), p. 126. This does not, of course, take account of the immeasurable but very real cost of the impact of huge uncertainty on those working in the NHS.

3 Ibid., p. 2.

4 Travis A (2012), 'Margaret Thatcher's role in plan to dismantle the welfare state revealed', *Guardian*, 28 December.

5 Clarke K (2008), *Rejuvenate or Retire? View of the NHS at 60*, Nuffield Trust.

6 Isard M and Kaffash J (2012), 'Revealed: One in five CCG board members have potential conflict of interest', *Pulse*, 21 December; Editors (2013), 'More than a third of GPs on commissioning groups have conflicts of interest, BMJ investigation shows', BMJ 346: f1569, 14 March, http://www.bmj.com/content/346/bmj.f1569?tab=citation.

7 The role of the honours system and diseases such as 'Knight Starvation' in corrupting the professions would be an interesting study.

8   See Jarman B (2012), 'When managers rule. Patients may suffer, and they're the ones who matter', editorial, *British Medical Journal*, 19 December.

9   Department of Health (2010), Reports commissioned by Ara Darzi on the NHS.

10 Many managers are as passionately committed to the NHS and its values as the best clinicians. I know this from personal experience of working with excellent managers – such as the dedicatee of my *Hippocratic Oaths*. They are placed under almost unbearable pressures, unlike the more self-focused and ambitious ones who will do whatever is necessary to prosper.

11 Leys C (2011), 'Friday lecture', Goldsmith's College, 8 April, based on Colin Leys and Stewart Player's book *The Plot Against the NHS*.

12 Owen D (2013), 'My plan to save the NHS', *Guardian*, 29 January.

13 This was first highlighted by the sociologist Emile Durkheim. It is discussed in Hippocratic Oaths, op cit.

14 See Horton R (2013), 'Offline: taking stock at the Royal College of Physicians', *The Lancet* 381: 710, 1 March.

15 Helm T and Campbell D (2013), 'Doctors cry foul at NHS "privatisation by stealth"', *Observer*, 2 March.

16 Multinationals circling with drooling chops around the NHS would hardly welcome doctors working together across institutions, disciplines and sectors with the aim of delivering the integrated service that an ageing patient population needs. The recent assault on clinical networks, described by Roger Boyle, the outgoing national director for heart disease and stroke (Boyle R (2013), 'Clinical networks work and shouldn't be disbanded', *BMJ* 346: 25, 2 February), is entirely consistent with a business model where the emphasis is on competition and not co-operation and doctors are to be discouraged from working together to develop optimal service configurations for the benefit of patients. Such anti-competitive collusions are to be resisted, just as the shift of care from hospitals to the community must be opposed by any foundation trust that is concerned to balance its books.

17 Gerada C (2012), *Guardian*, 3 February, quoted in Timmins (2012), *Never Again?*, p. 110.

18 Godlee F (2011), 'Dr Lansley's Monster', *BMJ* 342, 21 January.

19 Economist Ipsos MORI (2012), Issues Index, 21 February.

20 Leys (2011), 'Friday lecture'.

21 The Commonwealth Fund is a New York-based independent health policy unit. The findings of the study are summarised and analysed in Ingleby D, McKee M, Mladovsky P and Rechel B (2012), 'How the NHS measures up to other health systems', *BMJ* 344: e1079, 22 February.

22 *U.S. Health in International Perspective: Shorter Lives, Poorer Health* summarised in Editorial (2013), 'Wealth but not health in the USA', *The Lancet* 381 (9862): 177, 19 January.

23 Francis R (2013), 'The final report into the Mid-Staffordshire Foundation Trust'.

24 Briefing notes, National Health Service (Amended Duties and Powers) Bill 2013. See Appendix 2 of this book.

25 Press Association (2012), 'NHS shakeup spells "unprecedented chaos", warns *Lancet* editor', *Guardian*, 24 March, http://www.guardian.co.uk/society/2012/mar/24/nhs-shakeup-chaos-lancet

26 It will come as no surprise that a recent authoritative analysis has shown that competition between NHS providers drives down productivity. See Charlesworth A and Jones N (2013), *The Anatomy of Health Spending: A Review of NHS Expenditure and Labour Productivity*, Nuffield Trust.

1. Breaking the Public Trust

1 Lister J (2008), *The NHS After 60, for Patients or Profits?* Middlesex University Press.

2 Newman C (2011), 'FactCheck: The truth about the NHS reform bill myths', October 11, Channel 4 FactCheck, http://blogs.channel4.com/factcheck/factcheck-the-truth-about-the-nhs-reform-bill-myths/8160

3 Lister (2008), *The NHS After 60*, chapter 4.

4 One of the most enthusiastic was Tribal Newchurch management consultant Kingsley Manning, who hailed the White Paper proposals

as the 'denationalisation' of the NHS. Swindells M, Manning K (2010), '"Liberating the NHS" – the next turn in the cork screw?' Tribal Group, August, http://www.vac.org.uk/wordpress/wp-content/uploads/2010/08/LIBERATING-THE-NHS-POLICY-BRIEFING.pdf

5 Timmins N (2010), 'NHS reforms run full speed into unknown', *Financial Times*, 14 December, http://www.ft.com/cms/s/0/5c23dda2-07b7-11e0-a568-00144feabdc0.html#axzz2LCM7BNFo

6 Press Association (2011), 'NHS warned over higher efficiency savings', *Evening Standard*, 29 April, http://www.thisislondon.co.uk/standard/article-23945430-nhs-warned-over-higher-efficiency-savings.do

7 Collins N and Adams S (2012), 'More than half of NHS trusts rationing treatments', *Daily Telegraph*, 13 December, http://www.telegraph.co.uk/health/healthnews/9740922/More-than-half-of-NHS-trusts-rationing-treatments.html

8 McKinsey & Company (2009), 'Achieving world class productivity in the NHS, 2009/10-2013/14: Detailing the size of the opportunity', March, http://www.dh.gov.uk/prod_consum_dh/groups/dh_digitalassets/documents/digitalasset/dh_116521.pdf

9 Mooney H (2012), 'CCGs fail to engage "apathetic" GPs', *Pulse*, 14 September, http://www.pulsetoday.co.uk/ccgs-fail-to-engage-apathetic-gps/14596357.article

10 Lister J (2012), 'West London NHS bosses opt to advertise rather than consult', London Health Emergency press release, 12 September, http://www.healthemergency.org.uk/breakingnews.php

11 Lister J (2012), 'In defiance of the evidence: Conservatives threaten to "reform" away England's National Health Service', *International Journal of Health Services* 42 (1): 137–55.

12 n.a. (2011), 'Gateways using nurses to screen GP referrals', *Pulse*, 10 August, http://www.pulsetoday.co.uk/main-content/-/article_display_list/12511567/referral-gateways-using-nurses-to-screen-gp-referrals [14.8.]

13 NHS Commissioning Board (2012), Commissioning Support Bulletin –

Issue 5, 1 October, http://www.commissioningboard.nhs.uk/2012/10/01/cs-bulletin-issue5/

14 Lister J (2012), 'Saving the cancer, sacrificing the patient', National Health Action Party, December, http://www.healthemergency.org.uk/pdf/LondonHealthEmergencyResponsetoTSA-Dec2012.pdf

15 Department of Health (2005), 'A short guide to NHS Foundation Trusts', November, www.dh.gov.uk/nhsfoundationtrusts

16 Lister (2008), *The NHS After 60*, Middlesex University Press, pp. 154–9 and *passim*.

17 Gainsbury S (2010), 'Lansley signals FT removal from government balance sheet', *Health Service Journal*, 12 July, http://www.hsj.co.uk/news/finance/lansley-signals-ft-removal-from-government-balance-sheet/5017118.article

18 Reid J (2004), 'Statement in parliament on ministerial accountability for NHS Foundation Trusts', Hansard HC Deb, 11 October, c4WS, http://www.publications.parliament.uk/pa/cm200304/cmhansrd/vo041011/wmstext/41011m02.htm#41011m02.html_spmin0

19 Lister (2008), *The NHS After 60*, p. 238.

20 Public Accounts Committee (2013), 'Department of Health: the franchising of Hinchingbrooke Health Care NHS Trust and Peterborough and Stamford Hospitals NHS Foundation Trust', 28 January, www.parliament.uk/pac

21 Lister J (2013), 'Pure financial incompetence: the heavy price of PFI in the NHS in Eastern Region, UNISON Eastern Region, January, http://www.healthemergency.org.uk/pdf/PureFinancialIncompetence.pdf

22 Francis R (2013), *The Mid Staffordshire NHS Foundation Trust Public Inquiry*, February, http://www.midstaffspublicinquiry.com/report

23 Pollock AM, Price D, Roderick R, Treuherz T, McCoy D, McKee M and Reynolds L (2013), 'How the Health and Social Care Bill 2011 would end entitlement to comprehensive health care in England', *The Lancet* 26 January, http://www.thelancet.com, DOI:10.1016/S0140-6736(12)60119-6

24 Mehta C and Sher B (2013), 'OFT's first review of NHS Foundation Trust merger', *EU & Competition Briefing*, 10 January, Nabarro, http://www.nabarro.com/Downloads/EU-Competition-OFT's-first-review-of-NHS-Foundation-Trust-merger.pdf

25 Gainsbury S (2013), 'OFT may block basket case trust moves', *Health Service Journal*, 16 January, http://www.hsj.co.uk/opinion/oft-may-block-basket-case-trust-moves/5053585.article?blocktitle=Opinion&contentID=141

26 Calkin S (2013), 'CCP to consider acute services "merger" in Bristol', *Health Service Journal*, 11 February, http://www.hsj.co.uk/hsj-local/acute-trusts/university-hospitals-bristol-nhs-foundation-trust/ccp-to-consider-acute-services-merger-in-bristol/5054847.article

27 House of Commons (2013), *The National Health Service (Procurement, Patient Choice and Competition) Regulations 2013*, http://www.legislation.gov.uk/uksi/2013/257/pdfs/uksi_20130257_en.pdf

28 Timmins N (2007), 'Hospitals told to focus on profit centres', *Financial Times*, 12 March, http://www.ft.com/cms/s/0/21f089aa-d03e-11db-94cb-000b5df10621.html

29 Briggs H (2011), 'Planned 49% limit for NHS private patients in England', BBC News, 27 December, http://www.bbc.co.uk/news/health-16337904

30 Lister (2008), *The NHS After 60*, chapter 9.

31 HM Treasury (2012), PFI signed projects list, March, http://www.hm-treasury.gov.uk/ppp_pfi_stats.htm

32 Costello T (2012), 'NHS PFI firms avoid millions in tax', Bureau of Investigative Journalism, 4 September, http://www.thebureauinvestigates.com/2012/09/04/nhs-pfi-firms-avoid-millions-in-tax/

33 Lister J (2013), 'Lewisham: a test case for draconian powers', Campaigner's Diary, January, http://www.healthemergency.org.uk/diary.php

34 Clover B (2013), 'NHS earmarks £300m to put hospitals through failure regime', *Health Service Journal*, 18 January, http://www.hsj.co.uk/acute-care/nhs-earmarks-300m-to-put-hospitals-through-failure-regime/5053709.article

35 Dowler C (2012), 'Bennett moots PFI buyout for Peterborough', *Health Service Journal*, 11 December, http://www.hsj.co.uk/5052807. article?referrer=e2

2. Ready for Market

1   Feachem RGA, Sekhri NK, White KL, Dixon J, Berwick DM and Enthoven AC (2002), 'Getting more for their dollar: a comparison of the NHS with California's Kaiser Permanente', *BMJ* 19 January, http://www.bmj.com/content/324/7330/135

2   Talbot-Smith A, Gnani S and Pollock AM (2004), 'Questioning the claims from Kaiser', *British Journal of General Practice* 54 (503): 415–21, http://www.ncbi.nlm.nih.gov/pmc/articles/PMC1266198/

3   York GK (2000), 'Executives with white coats – managed-care medical directors', *New England Journal of Medicine* 342 (18), 4 May.

4   Price D, Pollock AM and Shaoul J (1999), 'How the World Trade Organisation is shaping domestic policies in health care', *The Lancet*, 27 November, http://www.thelancet.com/journals/lancet/article/PIIS0140-6736%2899%2911060-2/fulltext#article_upsell

5   Waitzkin H and Jasso-Aguilar R (2012), 'Health care and change: popular protest and building alternative visions of health systems at the end of empire', in Watson P (ed.), *Health Care and Globalisation*, Oxford: Routledge.

6   It should be pointed out that because the dominant form of MCO is the Health Maintenance Organisation, the terms are often used interchangeably. Another form of health care insurance vehicle in the US is the Preferred Provider Organisation (PPO), which is more likely to use negotiated fees for service payments with a specified network of providers.

7   A useful overview of the organisational formats in managed care is provided in a document by Gleave R (2009), 'Across the pond: lessons from the US on integrated healthcare', Nuffield Trust, January. The author was a 2007–08 Harkness Fellow in Health Care Policy based at Kaiser Permanente, and subsequently became director of patient experience

and planning for DoH England. He had previously been the NHS trust chief executive in Bath.

8   House of Commons (2003) Debates, 7 May, col. 714, http://www.publications.parliament.uk/pa/cm200203/cmhansrd/vo030507/debindx/30507-x.htm

9   The Commercial Directorate consisted of 190 people, no less than 182 of whom were 'interims' on secondment from the private sector. Among the companies introduced into large-scale NHS work were Netcare, Capio and Clincenta, as well as domestic brands such as BUPA and BMI. The directorate was disbanded in 2007, although its functions were transferred to regional commercial support units to help link private providers with NHS purchasers at the local level, much as troops fan out from a bridgehead once it has been consolidated.

10 British Medical Association (2007), 'Hospital consultants worth every penny, says BMA', press release, 22 November, http://web.bma.org.uk/pressrel.nsf/wall/2461950786BBA9F58025739A0043B614?OpenDocument

11 Dash P (2002), 'Plan B on the consultant contract', *Guardian*, 1 November, http://www.guardian.co.uk/society/2002/nov/01/health.publicservices

12 n.a. (2003), 'Stressed consultants eye NHS exit', *Healthcare Market News*, August.

13 Department of Health (2005), 'Creating a patient-led NHS: delivering the NHS Improvement Plan', 17 March, http://webarchive.nationalarchives.gov.uk/+/www.dh.gov.uk/en/Publicationsandstatistics/Publications/PublicationsPolicyAndGuidance/Browsable/DH_5112637

14 NHS National Leadership Network (2006), 'Strengthening local services: the future of the acute hospital', 21 March, https://www.eoe.nhs.uk

15 Carvel J (2005), 'The quiet revolutionary', *Guardian*, 15 June, http://www.guardian.co.uk/society/2005/jun/15/guardiansocietysupplement.interviews

16 Imison C (2012), 'NHS providers – is bigger better?', The King's Fund, 28 June, http://www.kingsfund.org.uk/audio-video/candace-imison-nhs-providers-%E2%80%93-bigger-better

17 Correspondence between the DoH and McKinsey during the period from October 2011 to February 2012 on the future viability of some hospitals was obtained following a request under the Freedom of Information Act by the Green Benches website. It revealed that: 'Days before the NHS Bill entered its final stages McKinsey and the DH were already discussing the merger of acute hospitals and the private financial takeover of whole hospitals.' As Imison was quick to point out in the above-mentioned King's Fund seminar, 'the evidence isn't great about mergers'.

18 House of Commons Public Accounts Committee (2012), 'Department of Health: securing the future financial sustainability of the NHS', 30 October.

19 Laurance J (2010), 'One NHS trust in five is in bad financial trouble – and Department of Health is failing to plan for bankruptcies', *Independent*, 30 October, http://www.independent.co.uk/life-style/health-and-families/health-news/one-nhs-trust-in-five-is-in-bad-financial-trouble--and-department-of-health-is-failing-to-plan-for-bankruptcies-8231603.html

20 See NHS Confederation 'The Practice' website at http://www.thepracticeplc.com/about-us

21 It's worth considering one of the ways in which the public relations aspect of the introduction of the highly controversial FESC was managed for the benefit of the public and medical profession, as it was a template that can be found in many other instances. Within days of the FESC announcement, a row out broke over potential conflicts of interest. Dr Mike Dixon, chair of the NHS Alliance, said that while a framework 'could help practice-based commissioning flourish', the private companies concerned 'must not themselves commission the care'. He continued: 'That's something we must never let happen'; there would be 'a major conflict of interest where a commissioning support team is also bidding to provide primary care'. Dr Dixon was, however, both the 'lead' figure for commissioning on Lord Darzi's new advisory board and a member of the advisory board for the US health care giant Humana. BUPA's medical director, Dr Natalie-Jane Macdonald, said conflicts of interest were

'everywhere', and 'not in any way limited to those with FESC contracts'. Dr Dixon's comments were a form of risk management, drawing attention away from the highly contestable nature of the FESC to a possible future conflict of interest between commissioning and service provision. In this way, the framework has been consolidated, the key statement being that the FESC 'framework can help practice-based commissioning flourish'.

22 The fourteen selected suppliers were: Aetna, Axa PPP, BUPA, CHKS, Dr Foster, Health Dialog Services Corporation, Humana, KPMG LLP, McKesson, McKinsey, Navigant Consulting, Tribal, UnitedHealth Europe and WG Consulting.

23 Support for this list of activities would come from various partners including PwC in alliance with, among others, The King's Fund and Cumberledge Connections; KPMG alongside UnitedHealth and the National Association for Primary Care; McKinsey with the RCGP and Ashridge Alliance; and others led by Ernst & Young and Capita. The remaining seven London CCGs were expected to sign up to the proposals as well.

24 n.a. (2008), 'Insurance firms eye top up opportunities', *Healthcare Market News*, December.

25 n.a. (2009), 'PCTs must provide clarity on top-ups', *Healthcare Market News*, March.

26 Royal College of General Practitioners (2008), 'Primary Care Federations – putting patients first: Feedback from the consultation', November, http://www.rcgp.org.uk/policy/rcgp-policy-areas/~/media/Files/Policy/A-Z%20policy/Primary_Care_Federations_consultation.ashx

27 According to a paper produced for the Nuffield Trust by Lawrence Casalino, the former vice president of a large US IPA, 'IPAs are networks of independent physicians who come together to hold a budget from insurance companies, but maintain their status as independent businesses. GP consortia will be much more like IPAs than like the Integrated Delivery Systems with which the NHS has been more familiar, such as Kaiser Permanente'.

28 The concept of integrated care now appears to be acting as a way of assuaging growing public hostility to the impending subjection of the NHS to a competitive free-for-all. During the listening pause called in May 2011 by Lansley during the debate over the health bill, 'integration' was promoted as far more politically acceptable, and the government immediately accepted the Future Forum's list of recommendations on the concept, though these recommendations were notably vague. Indeed Dr Bennett always reassured the private sector that the line on competition was non-negotiable. According to NHS Partners Network lobbyists, 'he has consistently taken the same line as us throughout'.

29 Featherstone H (2012), 'All together now: Competitive integration in the NHS', Policy Exchange, 1 November.

30 Caldwell-Nichols A and Pollard C (2012), 'Integrating care and preventing anti-competitive behaviour', The King's Fund, 18 September, http://www.kingsfund.org.uk/sites/files/kf/caldwell-nichols-pollard-monitor-integrating-care-preventing-anti-competitive-behaviour-kingsfund-sept12.pdf

31 Timmins N (2012), 'The aftermath of reform', *Health Service Journal*, 12 July.

32 Waitzkin H and Jasso-Aguilar R (2012), 'Health care and change'. Oxford: Routledge.

3. Parliamentary Bombshell

1 Timmins N (2012), *Never Again?: The Story of the Health and Social Care Act 2012 – A Study in Coalition Government and Policy*, London: The King's Fund.

2 Ham C (2013), 'The NHS in England in 2013', *BMJ* 346: e8634, http://www.bmj.com/content/346/bmj.e8634

3 British Medical Association (2010), 'BMA leader writes to the profession about "curate's egg" white paper', press release, 30 July, http://web.bma.org.uk/pressrel.nsf/wlu/SGOY-87UCEG?OpenDocument

4   Ireland T (2010), 'GP anger at being forced into consortia', *GP*, 22 July, http://www.gponline.com/News/article/1017168/GP-anger-forced-consortia/

5   The thirty-two-page list of organisations who submitted responses is available http://www.dh.gov.uk/prod_consum_dh/groups/dh_digitalassets/@dh/@en/@ps/documents/digitalasset/dh_123342.pdf

6   Ham C (2011), 'Competition in the NHS in England', *BMJ* 342: d1035, 14 February, http://www.bmj.com/content/342/bmj.d1035

7   The text of the document is available for download at: http://www.dh.gov.uk/en/Publicationsandstatistics/Publications/PublicationsPolicyAndGuidance/DH_122661

8   The text of the bill is available for download at: http://www.publications.parliament.uk/pa/cm201011/cmbills/132/11132.pdf

9   Delamoth T and Godlee F (2011) 'Dr Lansley's Monster', *BMJ* 342: 21 January, http://www.nhsca.org.uk/docs/bmjeditorial.pdf

10 Helm T (2011), 'Shirley Williams urges Lib Dems to fight Andrew Lansley's NHS plan', *Observer*, 12 March, http://www.guardian.co.uk/politics/2011/mar/12/shirley-williams-nick-clegg-nhs

11 Williams S (2011), opinion editorial, *The Times*, 28 February. For commentary on the piece, see Healthy Policy Insight (2011), 'Shirley, you can't be serious', 28 February, http://www.healthpolicyinsight.com/healthpolicyinsight.com/?q=node/972

12 Harris E (2011), 'Lib Dems stand strong against damaging NHS changes', *Guardian*, 4 April, http://www.guardian.co.uk/commentisfree/2011/apr/04/lib-dems-nhs-changes

13 Timmins (2012), *Never Again?*, p. 95.

14 Hansard (2011), House of Commons Debate, 4 April, http://www.publications.parliament.uk/pa/cm201011/cmhansrd/cm110404/debtext/110404-0002.htm#1104043000734

15 See the Department of Health 'NHS Future Forum members' web page, http://healthandcare.dh.gov.uk/nhs-future-forum-members/

16 Iacobucci G (2012), 'Lobbyists' document shows close working between

private sector and government over health bill', *BMJ* 345: e8111, 27 November, http://www.bmj.com/content/345/bmj.e8111

17 Munday J, Dalton T et al. (2011), 'Coalition's GP health reforms have the support of doctors responsible for seven million patients', *Telegraph*, 11 May, http://www.telegraph.co.uk/comment/letters/8505479/Coalitions-GP-health-reforms-have-the-support-of-doctors-responsible-for-seven-million-patients.html; the letter was submitted to the newspaper on 10 May and published in the following day's edition.

18 See this on video at http://vimeo.com/32529385

19 Holm T (2011), 'Shirley Williams plunges NHS reforms into fresh turmoil', *Observer*, 3 September, http://www.guardian.co.uk/politics/2011/sep/03/shirley-williams-nhs-reforms-turmoil

20 Owen P (2011), 'NHS reforms: House of Lords debate', *Guardian* live blog, 12 October, http://www.guardian.co.uk/society/joepublic/2011/oct/12/nhs-reforms-house-of-lords-debate-live

21 Chatterton J (2011), 'NHS legal review on duty to provide and competition – published today', 38 Degrees, 30 August, http://blog.38degrees.org.uk/2011/08/30/nhs-legal-review-on-duty-to-provide-competition-published-today/

22 The petition is archived at: http://epetitions.direct.gov.uk/petitions/22670

4. The Silence of the Lambs

1 British Medical Association (2010), 'BMA leader writes to the profession about "curate's egg" white paper', press release, 30 July, http://web.bma.org.uk/pressrel.nsf/wlu/SGOY-87UCEG?OpenDocument

2 n.a. (2010), 'Doctors urged not to panic by GPC', *Healthcare Republic*, 23 July, http://www.gponline.com/News/article/1017171/Doctors-urged-not-panic-GPC/

3 It is interesting to note how the language changed during the passage of the bill, shifting as it did to accommodate criticisms without ever altering the underlying principles involved. A classic example was

Notes • 249

changing 'Any Willing Provider', which had overtones of anyone with a mop and a bucket, to 'Any Qualified Provider', which had a much more professional ring to it. There was no actual change in the nature or requirements of 'providers' to accompany this change in terminology.

4   Moberly T (2010), 'GP commissioning to drive up clinical standards and productivity', *Healthcare Republic*, 22 July, http://www.gponline.com/News/article/1017823/GP-commissioning-drive-clinical-standards-productivity/

5   Jacques H (2012), 'Doctors reject calls to boycott Clinical Commissioning Groups', *BMJ*, 30 June, http://careers.bmj.com/careers/advice/view-article.html?id=20007724

6   n.a. (2010), 'More than just a brand: What does the white paper mean for the future of our NHS?', Unison, http://www.unison.org.uk/acrobat/19460.pdf

7   McVeigh T (2010), 'Fears grow over care of mentally ill as GPs say they don't want the job', *Observer*, 18 July, http://www.guardian.co.uk/society/2010/jul/18/mental-health-nhs

8   Ireland T (2010), 'GP anger at being forced into consortia', *Healthcare Republic*, 22 July, www.healthcarerepublic.com/GP/news/1017168/GP-anger-forced-consortia

9   LHE (2010), 'White Paper special issue', Autumn, http://www.healthemergency.org.uk/he-issues/he66.pdf

10   http://bma.org.uk/images/whitepaperbmabriefingdec2010_tcm41-202540.pdf

11   Timmins N (2012), *Never Again?: The Story of the Health and Social Care Act 2012 – A Study in Coalition Government and Policy*, London: The King's Fund, p. 79.

12   British Medical Association (2010), 'Government has not listened to concerns about NHS reforms, says BMA', press release, 15 December, http://web.bma.org.uk/pressrel.nsf/wall/0F763AA228DB6377802577FA004D7C36?OpenDocument

13 Peedell C and cosignatories (2011), 'Open letter to the BMA about the health White Paper', *BMJ*, 342: d7, 4 January, http://www.bmj.com/content/342/bmj.d7

14 For a 'live' blog account of the SRM meetings, see Ireland T (2011), 'BMA special representative meeting – full coverage', *GP Online*, 15 March, http://www.gponline.com/News/article/1059830/BMA-special-representative-meeting---Full-coverage/

15 Quinn I (2011), 'BMA members reject outright opposition to health bill in knife-edge vote', *Pulse*, 16 March, http://www.pulsetoday.co.uk/bma-members-reject-outright-opposition-to-health-bill-in-knife-edge-vote/11055484.article#.UVhuUTfm05U

16 British Medical Association (2011), 'Changes to health bill are significant, but success will depend on detail, says BMA', press release, http://web.bma.org.uk/pressrel.nsf/wall/3D7FA5D9CD89FC11802578AF004AA505?OpenDocument

17 n.a. (2011), 'Reaction: NHS Future Forum report', *Pulse*, 14 June, http://www.pulsetoday.co.uk/reaction-nhs-future-forum-report/12204537.article#.UQrDvPKqE5U

18 Chorley M (2011), 'A slice of Britain: Lib Dem guerrillas plot their next move', *Independent*, 19 June, http://www. Tariff is dropped as way to stop "cherry picking independent.co.uk/news/uk/politics/a-slice-of-britain-lib-dem-guerrillas-plot-their-next-move-2299731.html

19 Hawkes N (2012), 'Government abandons plans to use payments to prevent private providers selecting simplest cases', *BMJ* 345: 7878, 4 October, http://www.bmj.com/content/345/bmj.e6728

20 Watt N (2011), ' "NHS reform is safe" – Andrew Lansley makes private plea for Tory support', *Guardian*, 13 June, http://www.guardian.co.uk/politics/2011/jun/13/nhs-reform-andrew-lansley; Davis J (2011), 'This NHS U-turn was a fake', *Guardian*, Comment is free, 6 July, http://www.guardian.co.uk/commentisfree/2011/jul/06/andrew-lansley-health-bill

21 Iacobucci G (2011), 'Meldrum: time to move on', *Pulse*, 16 June, http://

www.pulsetoday.co.uk/meldrum-time-to-move-on/12205005.article#. UVCSBBmDvG4

22 Ibid.

23 Hansard (2011), Public Bill Committee, 28 June, col. 54, http://www. publications.parliament.uk/pa/cm201011/cmpublic/health/110628/ pm/110628s01.htm

24 Personal and confidential communications with the authors.

25 Kmietowicz Z (2011), 'BMA calls for amended health bill to be withdrawn', *BMJ* 343: d4701, 21 July, http://www.bmj.com/content/343/bmj.d4701

26 n.a. (2011), ' "Furious" Meldrum tells BMA: "Back me or sack me"', *Pulse*, 21 September, http://www.pulsetoday.co.uk/furious-meldrum-tells-bma-back-me-or-sack-me/12740915.article#.UVCcshmDvG4

27 Department of Health (2012), 'Developing commissioning support: towards service excellence', 2 February, http://www.commissioningboard. nhs.uk/wp-content/uploads/2012/01/NHSCBA-02-2012-8-Guidance-Developing-commissioning-support-Towards-service-excellence.pdf

28 Buckman L (2012), 'Letter from Laurence Buckman to Jeremy Hunt regarding contract changes', *Pulse*, 12 December, http://www.pulsetoday. co.uk/home/useful-resources/letter-from-laurence-buckman-to-jeremy-hunt-regarding-contract-changes/20001165.article

29 n.a. (2011), 'BMA opts for outright opposition after knife-edge vote', *Pulse*, 25 November, http://www.pulsetoday.co.uk/bma-opts-for-outright-opposition-to-health-bill-after-knife-edge-vote/13121234.article#. UVCf2xmDvG4

30 British Medical Association (2011), 'Health and Social Care Bill continues to cause chaos in the NHS, says BMA', press release, 7 December, http://web2.bma.org.uk/pressrel.nsf/wlu/RWAS-8PBD6C? OpenDocument&vw=wfmms

31 Nolan T (2012), 'Industrial action – winners and losers', BMJ Group Blogs, 25 June, http://blogs.bmj.com/bmj/2012/06/25/tom-nolan-industrial-action-winners-and-losers/

32 See http://www.rcseng.ac.uk/

33 Cooper C (2010), 'White Paper "once-in-a-lifetime" chance, says RCGP chief', GP Online, 7 October, http://www.gponline.com/News/article/1033076/White-Paper-once-in-a-lifetime-chance-says-RCGP-chief/

34 Campbell D (2010), 'Opponent of NHS reform driven by grim memories of 60s', *Guardian*, 19 November, http://www.guardian.co.uk/society/2010/nov/19/nhs-gp-leader-clare-gerada?INTCMP=SRCH

35 The programme aired on 23 February 2012. One transcript can be found at McCartney M (2012), 'Clare Gerada, Anna Soubry and "part time" doctors', Margaret McCartney Blog, 26 February, http://www.margaretmccartney.com/blog/?p=1341

36 Hansard (2011), Public Bill Committee, 30 June, col. 159, http://www.publications.parliament.uk/pa/cm201011/cmpublic/health/110630/pm/110630s01.htm

37 Davis J (2012), 'Calling our representatives to account over the bill', Hospital Dr, 6 February, http://www.hospitaldr.co.uk/blogs/dr-blogs/calling-our-representatives-to-account-over-the-bill

38 Rimmer A (2012), '98% of RCGP members call for health bill withdrawal', GP Online, 12 January, http://www.gponline.com/News/article/1111845/98-RCGP-members-call-Health-Bill-withdrawal/

39 Kasaraneni K (n.d.; closed 2013), 'Call for Mr Lansley to resign', e-petition, active through 24 January, archived at: http://epetitions.direct.gov.uk/petitions/27985

40 n.a. (2012), 'Lansley leans on Royal Colleges', Workers Revolutionary Party News Line, 28 January, http://www.wrp.org.uk/news/7221

41 Press Association (2012), 'Royal colleges will "continue dialogue" on reform', *Health Service Journal*, 27 January, http://www.hsj.co.uk/royal-colleges-will-continue-dialogue-on-reform/5040769.article

42 Personal correspondence (2011), with NHSCA, dated 17 August.

43 McKee M, Pollock AM, Clarke A, McCoy D, Middleton J, Raine R and Scott-Samuel A (2011), 'In defence of the NHS: why writing to the House of Lords was necessary', *BMJ*, 343: d6535, http://www.bmj.com/content/343/bmj.d6535

44 Beckford M (2011), 'Nearly 400 public health experts warn Lords to reject NHS reforms', *Telegraph*, 4 October, http://www.telegraph.co.uk/health/healthnews/8804619/Nearly-400-public-health-experts-warn-Lords-to-reject-NHS-reforms.html

45 Campbell D (2011), 'Labour promotes NHS "plan B" in last-ditch attempt to derail reforms', *Guardian*, 14 December, http://www.guardian.co.uk/society/2011/dec/14/labour-nhs-plan-b-reforms

46 n.a. (2012), 'Andrew Lansley heckled by June Hautot in NHS protest', *BBC News*, 20 February, http://www.bbc.co.uk/news/uk-17093082

47 Adams S and Mason R (2012), 'No. 10 health summit: Queen's former doctor "a political pawn"', *Telegraph*, 22 February, http://www.telegraph.co.uk/health/healthnews/9099065/No-10-health-summit-Queens-former-doctor-a-political-pawn.html

48 Timmins (2012), *Never Again?*, p. 24.

49 Ibid., p. 63.

50 Lepper J (2009), 'Tories back NAPC plan for GP budgets', *Healthcare Republic*, http://www.gponline.com/News/article/967465/Tories-back-NAPC-plan-GP-budge

51 Alessi C (2011), 'NHS shake-up will be better for docs, better for patients', *Sun*, 19 January, http://www.thesun.co.uk/sol/homepage/features/3358927/NHS-shake-up-will-be-better-for-doctors-and-better-for-patients.html

52 Ramesh R (2012), 'GP practice "offloaded vulnerable patients to save money"', *Guardian*, 31 May, http://www.guardian.co.uk/society/2012/may/31/gp-health-reform-cost-cut

53 Delgado M and Young A (2010), 'Police probe into missing £300k at Prince Charles' charity after bosses fail to file accounts', *Daily Mail*, 4 April, http://www.dailymail.co.uk/news/article-1263425/Police-yard-probe-missing-300k-Prince-Charles-charity.html

54 See http://www.nhsalliance.org/dr-michael-dixon/

55 n.a. (2011), 'Dr Johnny Marshall', *Pulse*, 5 May, http://www.pulsetoday.co.uk/14-dr-johnny-marshall/12200822.article#.UStYdzeqE5U

56 n.a. (2011), 'Dr James Kingsland', *Pulse*, 5 May, www.pulsetoday.co.uk/11-dr-james-kingsland/12200851.article#.USvbtDeqE5U

57 Naughton L (2012), 'BMA leadership dodge "slap on the wrist" over health bill opposition', *Management in Practice*, 23 May, http://www.managementinpractice.com/editors-pick/bma-leadership-dodge-%25E2%2580%2598slap-wrist%25E2%2580%2599-over-health-bill-opposition

58 Peedell C (2011), 'Further privatisation is inevitable under the proposed NHS reforms', *BMJ* 342: d2996, 17 May, http://www.bmj.com/content/342/bmj.d2996

59 Ham C (2011), 'If the NHS is doing well, why is it changing?', *Health Service Journal*, 18 November, http://www.hsj.co.uk/opinion/blogs/the-kings-fund-blog/if-the-nhs-is-doing-well-why-is-it-changing/5038117.blog

60 Torjesen I (2012), 'Public's satisfaction with NHS fell by 12% in 2011', *BMJ* 344: e4091, 12 June, http://www.bmj.com/content/344/bmj.e4091

61 McKee M, Cole K, Hurst L, Aldridge RW and Horton R (2011), 'The other Twitter revolution: how social media are helping to monitor the NHS reforms', *BMJ* 342: d948, 16 February, http://www.bmj.com/content/342/bmj.d948

62 Appleby J (2011), 'Does poor health justify NHS reform?', *BMJ* 342: d566, 27 January, http://www.bmj.com/content/342/bmj.d566

63 Personal communication with the authors.

64 Personal communication with the authors.

65 Personal communication with the authors.

66 Godlee F (2011), 'Dr Lansley's Monster', *BMJ* 342, 21 January, http://www.bmj.com/content/342/bmj.d408.long

67 Editors (2011), 'It's time to kill this Bill', *Lancet* 378: 9799, 8 October, http://www.lancet.com/journals/lancet/article/PIIS0140-6736%2811%2961555-9/fulltext

68 Timmins, *Never Again?*, p. 94.

69 Lilley R (2011), nhsManagers.net blog, 14 March, http://archive. constantcontact.com/fs065/1102665899193/archive/1104823784043.html

70 White C (2012), 'GPs are rejecting commissioning roles because of lack of interest', *BMJ* 344: e4369, 26 June, http://www.bmj.com/content/344/ bmj.e4369

71 White C (2012), 'BMA consults GMC about cash incentives to GPs to cut patient care', *BMJ* 345: e6445, 25 September, http://www.bmj.com/ content/345/bmj.e6445

72 Iacobucci G (2013), 'More than a third of GPs on commissioning groups have conflicts of interest, BMJ investigation shows', *BMJ* 346: f1569, 14 March, http://www.bmj.com/content/346/bmj.f1569

73 Macrae F (2013), 'GPs given control of NHS millions have ties to companies bidding for contracts', *Daily Mail*, 1 April, http://www. dailymail.co.uk/news/article-2302123/GPs-given-control-NHS-millions- ties-companies-bidding-contracts.html?ito=feeds-newsxml

74 Campbell D (2013), 'GPs' links to private healthcare firms spark fears of conflict of interest', *Guardian*, 14 March, http://www.guardian. co.uk/society/2013/mar/14/gps-clinical-commissioning-groups- private#history-link-box

75 White C (2012), 'Workload is rising and morale is falling among UK doctors, BMA survey shows', *BMJ*, 16 October, http://careers.bmj.com/ careers/advice/view-article.html?id=20009283

76 Jacque H (2012), 'Expect fireworks over the new GP contract', BMJ Group Blogs, 25 October, http://blogs.bmj.com/bmj/2012/10/25/ helen-jaques-expect-fireworks-over-the-new-gp-contract/

77 Hawkes N (2012), 'Government abandons plans to use payments to prevent private providers selecting simplest cases', *BMJ* 345: 7878, 4 October, http://www.bmj.com/content/345/bmj.e6728; Hudson B (2012), 'Why the NHS reforms sow seeds of confusion', *Guardian*, 4 December, http://www.guardian.co.uk/healthcare-network/2012/ dec/04/nhs-reforms-sow-seeds-confusion

78 White C (2012), 'CCGs swamped by red tape, warns NHS Clinical

Commissioners', 13 September, http://careers.bmj.com/careers/advice/view-article.html?id=20008824

5. A Failure of Politics

1   n.a. (1985), 'Knights bachelor', *London Gazette*, no. 50154, 15 June, p. 1, http://www.london-gazette.co.uk/issues/50154/supplements/1

2   The last meetings of the NHS Management Board were held in September 2011. See 'NHS Management Board: summaries of proceedings of scheduled meetings, Department of Health, http://www.dh.gov.uk/en/Publicationsandstatistics/Publications/PublicationsPolicyAndGuidance/DH_088441

3   For the full text of the act see http://www.legislation.gov.uk/ukpga/1990/19/contents/enacted

4   I have made this case on my blog. See West C (2011), 'The duty of a doctor: will you be able to trust your doctor?', Charles West, 14 October, http://west4mp.wordpress.com/2011/10/14/the-duty-of-a-doctor-will-you-be-able-to-trust-your-doctor/

5   The failures of PFI have been documented widely, both in this book; in research by Allyson Pollock, David Price and others; and in the media, including criticism from Andrew Lansley himself. See for example Gaffney D, Pollock AM, Price D, Shaoul J (1999), 'PFI in the NHS – is there an economic case?', *BMJ* 319: 116, 10 July, http://www.bmj.com/content/319/7202/116; Pollock A (2006), 'The exorbitant cost of PFI is now being cruelly exposed', *Guardian*, 26 January, http://www.guardian.co.uk/politics/2006/jan/26/publicservices.health; Rogers S and Ball J (2012), 'PFI contracts: the full list', *Guardian* DataBlog, 5 July, http://www.guardian.co.uk/news/datablog/2012/jul/05/pfi-contracts-list; Davies L and Mulholland H (2011), 'PFI schemes taking NHS trusts to brink of financial collapse, claims Lansley', *Guardian*, 22 September, http://www.guardian.co.uk/politics/2011/sep/22/pfi-schemes-nhs-trusts-brink-financial-collapse

6   See http://www.libdems.org.uk/latest_news_detail.aspx?title=Emergency_
    Motion:_Pakistan_Floods_-_carried&pPK=9796f229-9afd-44b7-af2a-
    7bb233558d7e

7   See http://www.libdems.org.uk/latest_news_detail.aspx?title=Emergency_
    Motion:_Trident_-_carried&pPK=9bd7bd33-84b7-4b43-83c5-
    c83666e6e95a

8   Adventure Capital Fund, 'About us', http://www.adventurecapitalfund.
    org.uk/content/view/14/29/

9   Bubb S (2011), 'At Cabinet!', Bubb's Blog, 14 June, http://bloggerbubb.
    blogspot.co.uk/2011/06/at-cabinet.html

10 Alessi C (2011), 'NHS shake-up will be better for docs, better for
    patients', *Sun*, 19 January, http://www.thesun.co.uk/sol/homepage/
    features/3358927/NHS-shake-up-will-be-better-for-doctors-and-better-
    for-patients.html

11 Campbell D (2012), 'Backers of NHS shake-up turn against Andrew
    Lansley's plans', *Guardian*, 7 February, http://www.guardian.co.uk/
    society/2012/feb/06/nhs-reforms-critics-andrew-lansley

12 Ramesh R (2012), 'GP practice "offloaded vulnerable patients to save
    money"', *Guardian*, 31 May, http://www.guardian.co.uk/society/2012/
    may/31/gp-health-reform-cost-cut

13 See, for instance, this transcript of a commentary piece given on US
    National Public Radio programme *Marketplace* in the late 1990s: http://
    www.drmccall.com/marketplace/marketplace02.html

14 Bubb S (2011), 'Of one mind!', Bubb's Blog, 7 June, http://bloggerbubb.
    blogspot.co.uk/2011/06/of-one-mind.html

15 Department of Health (2011), 'Government response to the NHS Future
    Forum report', CM 8113, The Stationery Office Ltd, June, available at
    http://www.official-documents.gov.uk/document/cm81/8113/8113.
    pdf

16 To send a motion to conference, we needed the formal support of either
    one local party or ten voting representatives. We had the support of two
    local parties and 217 voting reps.

17 See http://www.libdems.org.uk/autumn2011.aspx

18 For a fuller analysis of the Clegg/Williams letter, alongside the full text of the letter, see Reynolds L, Ruane S and McCoy D (2012), 'The Lib Dem conference and the NHS bill', Abetternhs's blog, 10 March, http://abetternhs.wordpress.com/2012/03/10/ldconf/. Another analysis was provided by Pollock A, Price D and Roderick P (2012), 'Statement by Professor Allyson Pollock, David Price and Peter Roderick in response to the Lib Dem "40 points" document', 9 March, http://www.allysonpollock.co.uk/administrator/components/com_article/attach/2012-03-09/Pollock_HouseOfLords_HSCB_StatementLibDem40Pts_09Mar12.pdf

19 As mentioned in chapter 3, it is standard practice in large government projects to use a risk register to record possible risks of the project and ways of mitigating such risks, and it is usual for such documents to be in the public domain. We know that a risk register on the possible risks of the NHS reforms has been in existence since September 2010, but it has never been released to the public.

20 To see the text of this emergency motion, numbered F19, visit http://www.libdems.org.uk/siteFiles/resources/docs/conference/2012-Spring/F19%20Protecting%20our%20NHS.pdf

21 The standard GP contract, dating from 1949 to the present day, has always been subject to changes, some negotiated by agreement and some imposed. It is called the GMS (General Medical Services) contract. Governments subsequent to the formation of the NHS have introduced PMS (Personal Medical Services) contracts and then APMS (Alternative Provider Medical Services).

22 These cases include $3.5 million paid to the US federal government, US Department of Justice (2004), 'United Healthcare Insurance agrees to pay US $3.5 million to settle fraud charges', press release, 13 December, http://www.justice.gov/opa/pr/2004/December/04_civ_788.htm; a total of $400 million paid ($50 million to New York State and $350 million to the American Medical Association), Goldstein A and Freifeld K (2009), 'UnitedHealth to settle over $400 million in manipulated payments to

doctors', Bloomberg, 15 January, http://www.kbla.com/Blog/2009/January/UnitedHealth_to_Settle_Over_400_Million_in_Manip.aspx; Hilzenrath D (2009), 'Research firm cited by GOP is owned by health insurer', *Washington Post*, 22 July, http://www.washingtonpost.com/wp-dyn/content/article/2009/07/22/AR2009072202216.html?hpid=topnews; and Parker Waichman LLP (2009), 'UnitedHealth Care reimbursement fraud victims lawsuits', http://www.yourlawyer.com/topics/overview/UnitedHealth_Care_Reimbursement_Fraud

23 Campbell D (2012), 'More NHS patients being treated by private firms, survey finds', *Guardian*, 19 November, http://www.guardian.co.uk/society/2012/nov/19/nhs-patients-treated-private-firms; Kelly E and Tetlow G (2012), 'Choosing the place of care: the effect of patient choice on treatment location in England, 2003-2011', Institute of Fiscal Studies and Nuffield Trust, 19 November, http://www.nuffieldtrust.org.uk/publications/choosing-place-of-care

24 Carvel J (2006), '£64bn NHS privatisation plan revealed', *Guardian*, 30 June, http://www.guardian.co.uk/society/2006/jun/30/health.politics

25 Department of Health (2006), 'Framework for procuring External Support for Commissioners (FESC): procurement at PCTs', various publications, http://webarchive.nationalarchives.gov.uk/+/www.dh.gov.uk/en/Managingyourorganisation/NHSprocurement/FESC/index.htm

26 Alliance on Lobbying Transparency (n.d.), 'Revolving door is unhealthy', http://www.lobbyingtransparency.org/15-blog/general/62-revolving-door-is-unhealthy

27 See the UnitedHealth Group website for a description of Stevens's and other executives' responsibilities, http://www.unitedhealthgroup.com/About/Executives.aspx

28 SmartHealthcare.com (2010), 'McKinsey leads DoH's consultancy roster', *Guardian* Professional, 15 September, http://www.smarthealthcare.com/department-health-mckinsey-consultancy-business-services-15sep10; Boffey D (2011), 'NHS reforms: American consultancy

McKinsey in conflict-of-interest row', *Observer*, 5 November, http://www.guardian.co.uk/society/2011/nov/05/nhs-reforms-mckinsey-conflict-interest

29   Woolf M (2005), 'The Monday interview: Nick Clegg: "The future of British politics will inescapably have to be liberal – with a small L"', *Independent*, 19 September. This quote was cited in various media during the debate of the Health and Social Care Bill, including in Ramesh R (2011), 'Why is the health and social care bill causing so much pain?', *Guardian* Comment Is Free, 6 October, http://www.guardian.co.uk/commentisfree/2011/oct/06/health-social-care-bill-andrew-lansley-nhs

30   Mulholland H (2011), 'NHS threatened by "disruptive" reforms, says Shirley Williams', *Guardian*, 28 February, http://www.guardian.co.uk/politics/2011/feb/28/nhs-threatened-reforms-shirley-williams

31   Williams S (2011), 'Why this flawed bill threatens the very future of the NHS', *Observer*, 4 September, http://www.guardian.co.uk/commentisfree/2011/sep/04/nhs-health-bill-andrew-lansley

32   The programme exposed Labour's Geoff Hoon, Stephen Byers, Patricia Hewitt, Baroness Sally Morgan and Margaret Moran and Conservative MP Sir John Butterfill. Channel 4 (2010), 'Politicians for hire', *Dispatches*, 22 March, episode summary http://www.channel4.com/programmes/dispatches/episode-guide/series-57/episode-1; a closer look at Stephen Byers was published on the Channel 4 blog Who Knows Who under the title 'MPs for sale: what will Byers influence?', http://whoknowswho.channel4.com/stories/MPs_for_sale%3A_What_will_Byers_influence_

33   See Social Investigations (2013), 'MPs financial links to companies involved in private healthcare', February (updated), http://socialinvestigations.blogspot.co.uk/p/mps-with-or-had-financial-links-to.html

34   Jowitt J (2012), 'Whitehall defends dual health roles of chairman of NHS watchdog', *Guardian*, 4 March, http://www.guardian.co.uk/politics/2012/mar/04/nhs-watchdog-ccp-lord-carter?INTCMP=SRCH. For an accounting of Lord Carter's interests see also, for example:

Corporate Watch (2011), 'Wolves cry wolf: selling competition in the NHS', 6 April, http://www.corporatewatch.org/?lid=3934 and Social Investigations (2012), 'One in six Labour peers have financial interests involved in private healthcare', 25 March, http://socialinvestigations. blogspot.co.uk/2012/03/one-in-six-labour-peers-have-financial.html

6. Hidden in Plain Sight

1   Leveson B (2011), 'Opening statement', Leveson Inquiry Part I, 14 November, http://www.levesoninquiry.org.uk/wp-content/uploads/2011/11/Transcript-of-Morning-Hearing-14-November-2011.txt

2   Penelope J (2011), 'Memo on Health and Social Care Bill', Parliament, http://www.publications.parliament.uk/pa/cm201011/cmpublic/health/memo/m121.htm

3   Timmins N (2012), *Never Again?: The Story of the Health and Social Care Act 2012 – A Study in Coalition Government and Policy*, London: The King's Fund, p. 38.

4   MacDonald V (2011), 'Leaked document shows how doctors can profit from NHS reform', Channel 4 News, 2 March, http://www.channel4.com/news/leaked-document-shows-how-doctors-can-profit-from-nhs-reform

5   Adetunji J (2011), 'Private company in talks with GPs to profit from patient spending savings', *Guardian* Professional, 2 March, http://www.guardian.co.uk/public-leaders-network/2011/mar/02/health-and-social-care?INTCMP=SRCH; Ramesh R (2011), 'NHS reform could see GP funds floated on stock market', *Guardian*, 2 March, www.guardian.co.uk/society/2011/mar/02/nhs-reform-surgeries-stock-market?INTCMP=SRCH

6   n.a. (2011), 'GP practices "could be partially floated on stock market" … making large profits for doctors', *Daily Mail*, 7 March, http://www.dailymail.co.uk/health/article-1362189/Andrew-Lansley-GP-practices-partially-floated-stock-market-profit.html

7   Boffey D and Helm T (2011), 'David Cameron's adviser says health reform

is a chance to make big profits', *Observer*, 14 May, http://www.guardian.co.uk/politics/2011/may/14/david-cameron-adviser-health-reform

8   n.a. (2011), 'Nick Clegg to oppose NHS competition regulator', BBC News, 18 May, http://www.bbc.co.uk/news/uk-politics-13435223

9   n.a. (2011), 'NHS reforms will mean big profits for private sector: astonishing confessions by David Cameron's own adviser', *Daily Mail*, 15 May, http://www.dailymail.co.uk/news/article-1387273/NHS-reforms-allow-private-sector-make-big-profits-says-David-Camerons-adviser.html

10   See, for example, Cohen T (2013), 'Cameron puts blame for NHS scandals on Labour: PM says party should take responsibility for "target-led agenda"', *Daily Mail*, 6 March, http://www.dailymail.co.uk/news/article-2289175/Cameron-puts-blame-NHS-scandals-Labour-PM-says-party-responsibility-target-led-agenda.html

11   Rose D (2012), 'The firm that hijacked the NHS: MoS investigation reveals extraordinary extent of international management consultant's role in Lansley's health reforms', *Mail on Sunday*, 12 February, http://www.dailymail.co.uk/news/article-2099940/NHS-health-reforms-Extent-McKinsey--Companys-role-Andrew-Lansleys-proposals.html#axzz2JvTqmM80 www.guardian.co.uk/society/2012/mar/27/gps-private-health-firm-shares

12   McKinsey's report 'From Austerity to Prosperity' by Sneader K, Roxburgh C, Dimson J, Baker G, et al., was released on 22 November 2010. For the full report or a copy of the press release, see http://www.mckinsey.com/insights/europe/from_austerity_to_prosperity_seven_priorities_for_uk. The *Telegraph* reprinted, nearly verbatim, the report's seven action points in the article, 'Seven priorities for long-term UK growth – McKinsey', *Telegraph*, 22 November, http://www.telegraph.co.uk/finance/economics/8149624/Seven-priorities-for-long-term-UK-growth-McKinsey.html. The preamble of the article gets the McKinsey report's title wrong, however, calling it 'From Prosperity to Austerity' – at least in the version available online in March 2013.

13   n.a. (2012), 'Andrew Lansley right man for NHS reform – Nick Clegg', BBC News, 14 February, http://www.bbc.co.uk/news/uk-politics-17011387

14 Campbell D (2012), 'GPs' shares in private healthcare firms prompt conflict of interest fears', *Guardian*, 27 March, www.guardian.co.uk/society/2012/mar/27/gps-private-health-firm-shares

15 n.a. (2010), 'Can GP power cure the NHS?', *Mirror*, 13 July, http://www.mirror.co.uk/news/uk-news/can-gp-power-cure-the-nhs-234990

16 MacDonald V (2011), '"Proof" government plans to privatise NHS?', Channel 4 News, 21 November, http://www.channel4.com/news/proof-government-plans-to-privatise-nhs

17 Watt H and Prince R (2010), 'Andrew Lansley bankrolled by private healthcare provider', *Telegraph*, 14 January, http://www.telegraph.co.uk/news/newstopics/mps-expenses/6989408/Andrew-Lansley-bankrolled-by-private-healthcare-provider.html

18 Watt H (2013), 'Two major Conservative donors appointed to government', *Telegraph*, 11 January, http://www.telegraph.co.uk/news/newstopics/mps-expenses/9794202/Two-major-Conservative-donors-appointed-to-government.html

19 Watt H, Prince R and Winnett R (2011), 'Wife of Health Secretary Andrew Lansley gave lobbying advice', *Telegraph*, 5 February, http://www.telegraph.co.uk/news/politics/8305506/Wife-of-Health-Secretary-Andrew-Lansley-gave-lobbying-advice.html

20 n.a. (2011), 'Health Secretary Andrew Lansley's wife comes under fire for discussing links with ministers on her company website', *Daily Mail*, 14 May, http://www.dailymail.co.uk/news/article-1386985/Health-Secretary-Andrew-Lansleys-comes-discussing-links-ministers-company-website.html#axzz2KUuu3E5U

21 Lyons J (2011), 'NHS reform leaves Tory backers with links to private healthcare firms set for bonanza', *Mirror*, 19 January, http://www.mirror.co.uk/news/uk-news/nhs-reform-leaves-tory-backers-105302

22 n.a. (2011), 'NHS reforms D-day: 40 peers have "financial interest" in NHS privatisation, Mirror investigation shows', *Mirror*, 12 October, http://www.mirror.co.uk/news/uk-news/nhs-reforms-d-day-40-peers-84917

23 n.a. (2012), 'NHS privatisation: compilation of financial and vested

interests', Social Investigations, 18 February, http://socialinvestigations.
blogspot.co.uk/2012/02/nhs-privatisation-compilation-of.html

24 n.a. (2011), 'NHS reforms D-day: 40 peers have "financial interest" in
NHS privatisation, Mirror investigation shows', *Mirror*, 12 October, http://
www.mirror.co.uk/news/uk-news/nhs-reforms-d-day-40-peers-84917

25 MacDonald V (2012), 'Government gives more ground on NHS reform',
Channel 4 News, 27 February, http://www.channel4.com/news/
government-gives-more-ground-on-nhs-reform

26 Poulton S (2012), 'Yes, we need to get our country working again. Sadly,
Workfare is not going to do it', *Daily Mail*, 29 February, http://poultonblog.
dailymail.co.uk/2012/02/index.html

27 Helm, T and Boffey D (2011), 'Lansley's ally on NHS reform faces
conflict of interest questions', *Guardian*, 29 May, http://www.guardian.
co.uk/politics/2011/may/29/lansley-ally-shareholding-lobby-firm

28 Rose D (2012), 'NHS fairness tsar urged to quit by doctors over "conflict
of interest" following £799,000 payment for U.S. private health giant', *Daily
Mail*, 4 March, http://www.dailymail.co.uk/news/article-2109907/NHS-
fairness-tsar-urged-quit-doctors-conflict-following-799-000-payment-U-
S-private-health-giant.html#axzz2KJKNNiWr

29 n.a. (2011), 'Andrew Lansley's NHS plans: still in good health?', Channel
4 News, 13 April, http://www.channel4.com/news/andrew-lansleys-nhs-
plans-still-in-good-health

30 n.a. (2010), 'Private health lobby out in force at Tory conference', SpinWatch,
4 October, http://www.spinwatch.org.uk/blogs-mainmenu-29/tamasin-
cave-mainmenu-107/5391-private-health-lobby-out-in-force-at-tory-
conference

31 Boffey D (2012), 'Jeremy Hunt in new row over bid to hire adviser from
private health sector', *Guardian*, 23 September, http://www.guardian.co.uk/
politics/2012/sep/23/jeremy-hunt-adviser-private-health?CMP=twt_gu

32 Robertson A (2012), 'Reform: A charity or a conduit for privatisation?',
openDemocracy, 20 September, http://www.opendemocracy.net/
ourkingdom/andrew-robertson/reform-charity-or-conduit-for-privatisation

33 See, for example, Haldenby A (2011), 'These "cuts" might do the NHS some good', *Telegraph*, 13 April, http://www.telegraph.co.uk/health/8448629/These-cuts-might-do-the-NHS-some-good.html; Haldenby A (2011), 'The NHS "listening exercise" is turning into a charade', *Telegraph*, 25 May, http://www.telegraph.co.uk/health/8535715/The-NHS-listening-exercise-is-turning-into-a-charade.html; Haldenby A (2011), 'The Coalition's NHS U-turn has been revealed', *Telegraph*, 26 May, http://www.telegraph.co.uk/health/8539660/The-Coalitions-NHS-U-turn-has-been-revealed.html; Haldenby A (2011), 'Why David Cameron's NHS speech will worry reformers', *Telegraph*, 6 June, http://www.telegraph.co.uk/health/8559873/Why-David-Camerons-NHS-speech-will-worry-reformers.html; Haldenby A (2011), 'One bad case does not discredit all private sector involvement in the NHS', *Telegraph*, 8 June, http://www.telegraph.co.uk/comment/letters/8562077/One-bad-case-does-not-discredit-all-private-sector-involvement-in-the-NHS.html; Haldenby A (2011), 'NHS reforms: the government is turning the clock back', *Telegraph*, 13 June, http://www.telegraph.co.uk/health/8573396/NHS-reforms-The-Government-is-turning-the-clock-back.html

34 n.a. (2012), 'The *Telegraph*, the think tank and a very dodgy business', Social Investigations, 2 August, http://socialinvestigations.blogspot.co.uk/2012/08/the-telegraph-think-tank-and-very-dodgy.html

35 Seddon N (2011), 'David Cameron is getting it wrong on NHS reform', *Telegraph*, 16 May, http://www.telegraph.co.uk/health/8516818/David-Cameron-is-getting-it-wrong-on-NHS-reform.html

36 Seddon N (2011), 'Why the NHS needs a regulator', *Telegraph*, 18 May, http://www.telegraph.co.uk/health/8521240/Why-the-NHS-needs-a-regulator.html

37 Huitson O (2012), 'How the BBC betrayed the NHS: an exclusive report on two years of censorship and distortion', openDemocracy, 27 September, http://www.opendemocracy.net/ourbeeb/oliver-huitson/how-bbc-betrayed-nhs-exclusive-report-on-two-years-of-censorship-and-distorti

38 Bishop D (2012), 'BBC's "extensive coverage" of the NHS bill', BishopBlog, 9 April, http://deevybee.blogspot.co.uk/2012/04/bbcs-extensive-coverage-of-nhs-bill.html

39 n.a. (2011), 'Lansley: My stroke influenced NHS reforms', Sky News, 17 April, http://news.sky.com/story/849524/lansley-my-stroke-influenced-nhs-reforms

40 Ramesh R (2012), 'Three-quarters of GPs want health and social care bill withdrawn, poll reveals', *Guardian*, 12 January, http://www.guardian.co.uk/society/2012/jan/12/gps-health-bill-withdrawn-poll

41 n.a. (2011), 'Andrew Lansley's NHS plans: still in good health?', Channel 4 News, 13 April, http://www.channel4.com/news/andrew-lansleys-nhs-plans-still-in-good-health

42 Montgomerie T (2011), 'The BBC has a monopoly and it's abusing it', ConservativeHome, 11 July, http://conservativehome.blogs.com/platform/2011/07/the-bbc-has-a-monopoly-and-its-abusing-it-says-timmontgomerie.html

43 See, for example: Editorial (2012), 'Don't let vested interests skew the NHS debate', *Independent*, 8 February, http://www.independent.co.uk/voices/editorials/leading-article-dont-let-vested-interests-skew-the-nhs-debate-6655115.html; Editorial (2012), 'Only the inefficient need fear NHS competition', *Telegraph*, 20 February, http://www.telegraph.co.uk/comment/telegraph-view/9093565/Only-the-inefficient-need-fear-NHS-competition.html; Comment (2011), 'Don't let ideology sink NHS reform', *Daily Mail*, 27 December, http://www.dailymail.co.uk/debate/article-2079196/MAIL-COMMENT-Don-t-let-ideology-sink-NHS-reform.html

44 Ipsos MORI (2011), 'Doctors are most trusted profession – politicians least trusted', 27 June, http://www.ipsos-mori.com/researchpublications/researcharchive/2818/Doctors-are-most-trusted-profession-politicians-least-trusted.aspx

45 Newton K (2006), *May the Weak Force Be with You: The Power of the Mass Media in Modern Politics*, Oxford: Blackwell Publishing Ltd.

46 Negrine R (1994) *Politics and the Mass Media in Britain*, 2nd ed., London: Routledge, p. 66.

7. From Cradle to Grave

1   'Report of the Inter-Departmental Committee on Social Insurance and Allied Services' (the 'Beveridge Report'), Cmnd 6404, London: HMSO.

2   This account of the origins of the NHS is adapted from a paper that we at the Health Policy & Health Services Research Unit of the School of Public Policy, University College London, prepared in 2002 for Unison, 'What's good about the NHS: and why it matters who provides service', April, http://www.unison.org.uk/acrobat/B325.pdf

3   National Health Service Act 1946. While the text is not currently available online via the UK government, it can be read at the website of the *Pittsburgh Post-Gazette*, which cited it during the debates over the US Patient Protection and Affordable Health Care Act, which President Obama signed into law in March 2010. See http://old.post-gazette.com/pg/10119/1054305-114.stm

4   Pollock AM (2004), *NHS plc: The Privatisation of Our Health Care*, 2nd ed., London: Verso.

5   Department of Health (2010), 'Liberating the NHS: regulating providers', 15 December, p. 3, http://webarchive.nationalarchives.gov.uk/+/www.dh.gov.uk/en/Consultations/Liveconsultations/DH_117782

6   Conservative Party (2011), 'Modernising the NHS: the Health and Social Care Bill', http://www.conservatives.com/News/News_stories/2011/01/Modernising_the_NHS.aspx

7   House of Lords (2011), Health and Social Care Bill, HL Bill 92, http://www.publications.parliament.uk/pa/bills/lbill/2010-2012/0119/2012119.pdf

8   Howe E (2011), Communication to Baroness Jay of Paddington, 'Health and Social Care Bill: 18th report of session 2010–12', paragraphs 8 and

25, 10 October, Appendix 2, http://www.publications.parliament.uk/pa/ld201012/ldselect/ldconst/240/240.pdf

9   House of Lords Select Committee on the Constitution (2011), 'Health and Social Care Bill: Follow-up', HL Paper 240, Appendix 2: correspondence, 20 December, www.publications.parliament.uk/pa/ld201012/ldselect/ldconst/240/24002.htm

10   This section is based on the following briefings and articles: Pollock AM, Price DP, Roderick P (2012), 'How the Health and Social Care Bill 2011 would end entitlement to comprehensive health care in England', *The Lancet* 6736: 12, 26 January, http://www.lancet.com/journals/lancet/article/PIIS0140-6736%2812%2960119-6/fulltext; Pollock AM, Price D and Roderick P (2012), 'Health and Social Care Bill 2011: A legal basis for charging and providing fewer health services to people in England', *BMJ* 344: e1729, 8 March, http://www.bmj.com/content/344/bmj.e1729; Pollock AM and Price D (2011), 'How the Secretary of State for Health proposes to abolish the NHS in England', *BMJ* 342: d1695, 22 March, http://www.bmj.com/content/342/bmj.d1695; Pollock AM, Price D, Roderick P and Treuherz T (2011), 'Health and Social Care Bill 2011, House of Lords Committee stage, briefing note 6 clause 10', 11 November, http://www.allysonpollock.co.uk/administrator/components/com_article/attach/2011-11-11/AP_2011_Pollock_HouseOfLordsBriefing6C10_11Nov11.pdf; Pollock A, Price D, Roderick P, Treuherz T, McCoy D, McKee M, Reynold L and Winyard G (2011), 'Health and Social Care Bill 2011, House of Lords report stage, briefing note 10: red lines for peers on the NHS bill', 9 January, http://www.allysonpollock.co.uk/administrator/components/com_article/attach/2012-01-09/20120109-AP_2012_Pollock_HouseOfLordsBriefing10_C1412_09Jan12.pdf; Pollock AM, Price D, Roderick P and Treuherz T (2011), 'Health and Social Care Bill, briefing on clause 1', 22 October, http://www.allysonpollock.co.uk/administrator/components/com_article/attach/2011-10-26/AP_2011_Pollock_HouseOfLordsBriefingC1__22Oct11.pdf; Pollock AM, Price D, Roderick P and Treuherz T (2012), 'Health and Social Care Bill, briefing

note 12, Earl Howe's response to the Constitution Committee's follow-up report and his letter dated 12 January', http://www.allysonpollock.co.uk/administrator/components/com_article/attach/2012-01-17/Pollock_HouseOfLords_HSCB_Briefing12_HoweLetter_17Jan12.pdf

11 Department of Health (2011), 'Healthy lives, healthy people: update and way forward', July, Cm 8134, http://www.official-documents.gov.uk/document/cm81/8134/8134.pdf

12 Clover B (2013), 'Exclusive: Nearly 50 trusts "have no independent future"', *Health Service Journal*, 25 March, http://www.hsj.co.uk/news/policy/exclusive-nearly-50-trusts-have-no-independent-future/5056524.article?blocktitle=Latest-News&contentID=8803

13 Pollock AM, Price DP, Roderick P, Treuherz T, McCoy D, McKee M and Reynolds L (2012), 'How the Health and Social Care Bill 2011 would end entitlement to comprehensive health care in England', *The Lancet* 379 (9814), 4 February, http://www.lancet.com/journals/lancet/article/PIIS0140-6736%2812%2960119-6/fulltext

14 Pollock AM, Price D and Roderick P (2012), 'Health and Social Care Bill 2011: a legal basis for charging and providing fewer health services to people in England', *BMJ* 344: e1729, 8 March, http://www.bmj.com/content/344/bmj.e1729

15 Ramesh R and Lawrence F (2012), 'Virgin Care to take over children's health services in Devon', *Guardian*, 12 July, http://www.guardian.co.uk/society/2012/jul/12/virgin-care-children-nhs-devon

16 Adams S (2012), 'NHS patients to be treated by Virgin Care in £500m deal', *Telegraph*, 20 March, http://www.telegraph.co.uk/health/health-news/9176733/NHS-patients-to-be-treated-by-Virgin-Care-in-500m-deal.html

17 n.a. (2012), 'Suffolk Community Healthcare: 66 frontline posts to go, says union', BBC News, 19 November, http://www.bbc.co.uk/news/uk-england-suffolk-20395749

18 Hellowell M and Pollock AM (2009), 'The private financing of NHS hospitals: politics, policy and practice', *Economic Affairs* 29, 3 March: 13–19.

19 Plimmer G (2012), 'Virgin keeps a low profile in healthcare', *Financial Times*, 9 December, http://www.ft.com/cms/s/0/087158f6-3f0a-11e2-9214-00144feabdc0.html#axzz2IsoYpv5t

20 Royal Commission on the National Health Service (1979), Report, Cmnd 7615, London: HM Stationery Office, http://www.sochealth.co.uk/national-health-service/royal-commission-on-the-national-health-service-1979/

21 Department of Health (2012), 'Securing the future financial sustainability of the NHS', Sixteenth Report of Session 2012–13, House of Commons, Committee of Public Accounts, http://www.publications.parliament.uk/pa/cm201213/cmselect/cmpubacc/389/389.pdf

22 Dilnot A (2012), Letter to Right Hon. Jeremy Hunt MP, 4 December, http://www.statisticsauthority.gov.uk

23 McKinsey and Company (2009), 'Achieving world class productivity in the NHS 2009/10 – 2013/14: detailing the size of the opportunity', March, see http://www.rightcare.nhs.uk/index.php/2010/07/achieving-world-class-productivity-in-the-nhs-200910-201314-detailing-the-size-of-the-opportunity/

24 Pollock A, Price D and Harding-Edgar L (2013), 'Briefing paper – the NHS reinstatement bill', openDemocracy, January, http://www.opendemocracy.net/ournhs/allyson-pollock-david-price-louisa-harding-edgar/briefing-paper-nhs-reinstatement-bill

25 Gaynor M, Laudicella M and Propper C (2012), 'Can governments do it better? Merger mania and hospital outcomes in the English NHS', CMPO working paper 12/281, http://www.bristol.ac.uk/cmpo/publications/papers/2012/wp281.pdf

26 Quoted in Royal Commission on the National Health Service (1979).

27 Owen D (2013), 'A bill to re-instate the NHS?', openDemocracy, 28 January, http://opendemocracy.net/ournhs/david-owen/bill-to-re-instate-nhs

28 To read the NHS reinstatement bill text and explanatory notes, see http://www.opendemocracy.net/ournhs/david-owen/nhs-reinstatement-bill-text-and-explanatory-notes

8. Stop Press: The Final Betrayal

1   Lansley A (2012)' Letter 'To leaders of all prospective CCGS', 16 February, http://falseeconomy.org.uk/files/lansley-ccg.pdf

2   Cutcher N and Reynolds L (2013), 'The NHS as we know it needs a prayer', openDemocracy, 19 February, http://www.opendemocracy.net/ournhs/nicola-cutcher-lucy-reynolds/nhs-as-we-know-it-needs-prayer

3   The text of section 75 is available at http://www.legislation.gov.uk/ukpga/2012/7/section/75/enacted

4   n.a. (2013), 'Lucy Reynolds talks to Jill Mountford', video, March, http://www.youtube.com/watch?v=OkTnCtg_Omk

5   Hansard (2013), House of Lords debate, 24 April, column 1496, http://www.publications.parliament.uk/pa/ld201213/ldhansrd/text/130424-0003.htm

6   Molloy C (2013), Twitter comment, 11 March, https://twitter.com/carolinejmolloy/status/311187913297760257

7   British Medical Association (2013), 'Lords debate motion to annul Section 75 regulations, 24 April 2013', http://bma.org.uk/working-for-change/the-changing-nhs/competition-and-choice/choice-and-competition/section-75-briefing

8   Hansard (2013), House of Lords debate, 24 April, column 1482, http://www.publications.parliament.uk/pa/ld201213/ldhansrd/text/130424-0002.htm#13042483000766

9   Hansard (2013), House of Lords debate, 24 April, column 1509, http://www.publications.parliament.uk/pa/ld201213/ldhansrd/text/130424-0003.htm

10 Hansard (2013), House of Lords debate, 24 April, column 1497, http://www.publications.parliament.uk/pa/ld201213/ldhansrd/text/130424-0003.htm

11 Warner N (2013), 'Warner: Why I will be voting for NHS competition regulations', *Health Service Journal*, 23 April, http://www.hsj.co.uk/opinion/warner-why-i-will-be-voting-for-nhs-competition-regulations/5057786.article

Afterword

1   n.a. (2012), 'NHS privatisation: compilation of financial and vested interests', Social Investigations, 18 February, http://socialinvestigations. blogspot.co.uk/2012/02/nhs-privatisation-compilation-of.html

2   Lawrence F (2013), 'Private contractor fiddled data when reporting to NHS, says watchdog', *Guardian*, 7 March, http://www.guardian.co.uk/society/2013/mar/07/private-contractor-data-nhs-watchdog?CMP=twt_gu

3   Cadigan P (2013), 'Taking stock at the Royal College of Physicians', *The Lancet* 281: 9871, 6 March, http://www.thelancet.com/journals/lancet/article/PIIS0140-6736%2813%2960322-0/fulltext

4   Horton R (2013), 'Offline: taking stock at the Royal College of Physicians', *The Lancet* 381: 9868, 2 March, http://www.thelancet.com/journals/lancet/article/PIIS0140-6736%2813%2960357-8/fulltext

5   Kaucher L (2013), 'The real force behind the NHS Act – the EU/US trade agreement', 19 February, www.opendemocracy.net/ournhs/linda-kaucher/real-force-behind-nhs-act-euus-trade-agreement

6   Calkin S (2013), 'Local Healthwatch "bound and gagged"', *Health Service Journal*, 11 January, http://www.hsj.co.uk/news/policy/local-healthwatch-bound-and-gagged/5053509.article

7   Katwala S (2013), 'The NHS: even more cherished than the monarchy and the army', *New Statesman*, 14 January, http://www.newstatesman.com/politics/2013/01/nhs-even-more-cherished-monarchy-and-army

8   Edmondson N (2012), 'Cameron's NHS reforms: "Opposition inevitable but rarely unbeatable"', *International Business Times*, 1 February, http://www.ibtimes.co.uk/articles/291078/20120201/cameron-blair-nhs-reforms.htm

About the Contributors

Dr Jacky Davis is a consultant radiologist at the Whittington Hospital in north London, member of the BMA Council, co-chair of the NHS Consultants' Association and a founder member of the campaign Keep Our NHS Public.

Oliver Huitson is co-editor of the British section of openDemocracy. He contributed the chapter 'The privatisation of our governance' to *Public Service on the Brink* and is reading for a Masters in Politics and Government at Birkbeck, University of London.

Dr John Lister has since 1984 been director of London Health Emergency, a pressure group fighting cuts, closures, privatisation and PFI throughout the NHS. He is the author of *Health Policy Reform*, *The NHS After 60* and *Europe's Health for Sale*. London Health Emergency was founded in the autumn of 1983 as an umbrella organisation for local campaigns defending hospitals in the capital against closure.

Ken Loach's most recent documentary, *The Spirit of '45*, celebrates the creation of Britain's welfare state.

Stewart Player is a public policy analyst with extensive experience of studying the NHS. He is co-author, with Colin Leys, of *The Plot Against the NHS*.

Allyson M. Pollock is professor of public health research and policy at Queen Mary, University of London. She set up and directed the Centre for International Public Health Policy at the University of Edinburgh from 2005 to 2011, and prior to that she was head of the Public Health Policy Unit at UCL. She is the author of *NHS plc*.

David Price is a senior research fellow in the Global Health, Policy and Innovation Unit at Queen Mary, University of London.

Prof. Raymond Tallis was for many years professor of geriatric medicine at the University of Manchester and is chair of Healthcare Professionals for Assisted Dying and a clinical neuroscientist. An acclaimed philosopher, he is the author of *Hippocratic Oaths*, *The Kingdom of Infinite Space* and *Aping Mankind*, among many books, and a frequent contributor to *The Times*.

Dr Charles West was the Liberal Democrat parliamentary candidate for Shrewsbury in 2010. He is a retired general practitioner.

Dr David Wrigley is an NHS general practitioner based in Lancashire. He is a member of the BMA General Practitioners Committee and previous member of the BMA Council. He passionately believes in the NHS and its importance as a fair, equitable, publicly funded, publicly provided and publicly accountable service.